Once
I
Was
Blind…

Gregg A. Milliken

ISBN 978-0-578-01381-7

Acknowledgments

I want to extend my personal and sincere thanks to:

Dr. Melvin Gerber —for opening the door for me to regain my eyesight and providing me with much needed resources in my time of need.

Dr. Clive Sell—for performing the surgery that changed my life and returning to me the gift of my eyesight. May God always bless you.

The Insulet Corporation—for bringing the OmniPod insulin pump to the market and allowing me, and countless others that suffer from this disease, to control my diabetes with no wires and amazing ease.

The City of Phoenix—for providing me with employment despite my disease and providing top-grade medical insurance.

American Diabetes Association—for everything this organization does to raise awareness of diabetes, support those of us that suffer from it, and for promoting my endeavors.

Juvenile Diabetes Research Foundation International—for their endless dedication to finding a cure.

Debbie McWhorter, my beloved mother—for helping me accept my disease and for always loving me and caring for me and supporting my endeavors.

My brothers and sisters in Jesus Christ—for providing an endless stream of support and encouragement.

My precious children Sierra, Ericca, Tristen, and Ava—for bringing me endless joy and for your loving understanding of the dynamics of my disease.

And, most of all, to my beautiful wife—thank you for all of your hard work, faithfulness, and for always believing in me.

Table of Contents

Introduction

The last trophy that I received was from the Ford Punt, Pass, and Kick Competition in 1971. It still sits on my television today as a reminder of my pre-diabetic days: shiny, perfect, and blemish-free. Before I was diagnosed, I was a perfectly normal child. I lived free, played hard, and was oblivious to disease. Before I was diagnosed, I was also a fairly decent sized young man. I felt very healthy. I had limitless stores of energy. My biggest worries were how I was going to build more muscle and how I was going to become a professional football player. My father's dream was for me to become a professional football player and I was heading toward that dream one pass at a time.

I remember getting that trophy as if it were just yesterday. As I sit here in my living room and stare at it, it stares back at me with a shiny perfection that is almost gone from my memory. It stares back at me with the reminders of a disease free life. That trophy reminds me of what it was like not to need insulin injections every day. It reminds me of what it was like not to worry about where my blood glucose level is at least six times a day. It reminds me of not worrying about the destruction diabetes is having on my body: the destruction on my mental health, my spiritual health, my physical health. It reminds me of how simple life was when I was oblivious to disease and insulin and glucose. It also reminds me of another thing: this disease can be overcome. It can be overcome through discipline. It can be overcome through faith in God. It can be overcome through diet and lifestyle and determination.

Before I developed this disease, I did not crave sweets. Before I developed this disease, I could eat whatever I wanted. I was still a child that could eat a candy bar and just enjoy it. I had the freedom that every other child had. I did not have to have discipline – the discipline that everyone fears if they get this disease.

Before I was diagnosed, I did not truly understand the true meaning of *disease*. Up until that point, I only understood sickness. Sickness was something that could be fixed. I was no stranger to sickness. I suffered from every ailment that is normal during childhood: strep throat, chicken pox, flu. I viewed sickness through the eyes of a child. I viewed sickness as a mere inconvenience that caused me to miss school and be pampered by my parents until the sickness was over. It never occurred to me that a sickness might exist that doctors, antibiotics, my parents and a few days in bed watching cartoons could not cure. It never occurred to me, even when I first heard the word "diabetes", that I would be learning through experience the difference between *sickness* and *disease.*

As I grew older, I noticed that a large number of people began to follow healthier diets as the United States seemed to be overcome with an epidemic of diabetes. As I watched this epidemic evolve, I began to feel that God had something special in store for my life. I felt that God made me special, not diseased. I realized that everyone I knew now knew someone with diabetes. I watched everyone around me try to change their diet to ensure that they did not develop my disease. I watched everyone around me, as the United States has become more aware of diabetes, live in fear of waking up every day to my reality. No one wants to give themselves six to eight injections a day. No one wants to rely on an insulin pump. No one wants to prick their fingers six to eight times a day. No one wants to deny themselves the luxury of a sweet dessert. No one wants to go to bed at night and wonder if their blood glucose levels will stay high enough to keep them alive overnight. No one wants this horrible disease. No one wants the disease that has plagued my life since I was nine years old.

Chapter One

Becoming "Diabetic"

Being diagnosed with diabetes is traumatic, to say the least. It is difficult to accept at any age that you have an incurable disease and as a child it is almost impossible. But even at nine years old, I realized that I had a long road ahead of me. Even at nine years old, I realized that my life was about to change forever.

The year was 1972. I lived in Flagstaff, Arizona. Up until that year I enjoyed a normal childhood. I had chicken pox that year, just like everyone else. I played football alongside my friends. I enjoyed the freedom of being a child and living my young life to the fullest. That was the year, however, that I also began to notice some changes in my body that came about rather quickly. I began to notice that I made unlimited trips to the restroom. I began to notice that I was thirsty all the time. I was not just thirsty: thirst was a normal part of life living in the Arizona desert. I was constantly parched to the point that I began to feel as if my thirst was impossible to quench. I also began to crave sweets. I did not just crave sweets like every other kid that begs for a candy bar or cake for dessert. I craved sweets with a shakiness and sickness that I had never experienced before and that I could not explain. I began to feel like I NEEDED sugar or I simply was not going to make it through the day. I began to realize, even at nine years old, that this was not normal.

The day I will never forget is the day that I was diagnosed with diabetes. That was the day that my life changed completely. That was the day I changed from a normal child to a "diabetic" child. On that particular day, I remember arriving home from school and desperately craving something sweet. My entire body was shaking and I was beginning to feel nauseous. I was frantically searching the kitchen for sugar when I finally discovered two bags of Hershey's kisses hidden behind some cans in the pantry. I loved Hershey's kisses. (So did my mother, which is why they were hidden behind the canned food.) Just as I finished that second bag – standing in front of the pantry door surrounded by what seemed like hundreds of tiny silver foils - I began to feel sick. Not the kind of sick you feel when you eat too much candy: it was a different kind of sick. It was a sickness that I had never felt before. I began to feel a sickness that brought me to my knees in the kitchen floor. This new sickness was a sickness that robbed me of my ability to speak or move. This new sickness caused my body to sweat profusely and seize uncontrollably. This new sickness caused my mother, a nurse, to scream when she entered the kitchen. The last sound that I heard before I awoke in the hospital was the panicked scream that escaped from my mother when she found me.

I do not remember the ride to the hospital. The last thing that I recall before waking in the hospital to my parents and a doctor speaking softly in a corner is losing consciousness in the kitchen floor to the sound of my mother screaming. As the fuzz was leaving my brain, I suddenly realized that I was in the hospital. I tried to focus on what my parents and the doctor were discussing so quietly, but to no avail. I looked down at my arms and noticed that one of them had an IV that was attached to a clear bag that hung just over my head. I began to wonder if this was reality or if I was dreaming. Once the three of them finally looked over and noticed that I was awake, the doctor walked over and gently took my hand. He smiled, told me that I would be "fine", and then told me that I had diabetes. At the time, I did not even know what that meant. "Diabetes" was a strange word. Out of all the words that I had ever heard in my entire life, I could not ever remember hearing this one. I remember thinking that it must be something awful, because every time the doctor said it, it made my mother cry. I must have looked as confused as I felt, because the doctor began to go into this crazy explanation of how I could no longer eat sugar like I had in my kitchen that day and that I would have to take injections everyday for the rest of my life. About half way through this ridiculous dialogue I convinced myself that I had to be dreaming. I was having a hard time comprehending exactly what this doctor was telling me. It seemed impossible that innocent little Hershey's kisses had landed me in the hospital. And injections? I had never had to take injections before. Well, of course I was vaccinated as a baby and before I began kindergarten, but I was sure that I did not need any more vaccines until I was at least eleven years old. I was about to explain to this kind, yet crazy doctor that I was only nine years old and I did not need any more vaccines yet when a nurse came in and handed me an orange and a syringe. My mind was absolutely spinning. That doctor was not talking about vaccines. This doctor was really telling me that I had to give myself injections everyday for the rest of my life. As I just sat there and held this orange and this syringe, this smiling nurse explained to me that I had to "practice" giving injections to this orange because next I would be giving injections to myself. What?? Was she really talking to me? Did I just wake up to this crazy nurse telling me to give this orange an injection? Why did I need this injection again? Did I catch a disease from poisoned Hershey's kisses? I had heard about people getting sick from poisoned food, but I could not believe that this was really happening to me. And why for the rest of my life? I thought that food poisoning went away after a few days. I gave myself a little pinch which brought me to the reality of the fact that I was awake and this nurse was really talking to me. I just could not believe what I was hearing. I remember just looking at this orange and this syringe in my hands and wondering exactly what I had missed while I was unconscious. The shock of it all was almost overwhelming. I finally asked the doctor is this was food poisoning. He laughed and told me again that I had *diabetes*. He told me that some doctors call it "sugar diabetes" because your body can no longer use sugar the way that it is supposed to use it. I tried to understand, but it was all so strange and so surreal. I remember the blur of nurses telling me: "its okay" and "its really not so bad." Then they told me that I will be giving myself injections for the rest of my life and that I could not eat two bags of Hershey's kisses ever again or I would probably die. Die? I still could not believe that all of this was happening because I ate Hershey's kisses. I loved Hershey's kisses. Although I loved Hershey's kisses, I absolutely hated needles. I did not just hate needles, I was absolutely terrified of them. I was one of those children that could not even look if I knew that a needle was coming. I had to close my eyes and hold my breath the last time that I got my vaccines so that I would not just freak out. Now I was being told that *I* would be giving myself injections every day for the rest of my life. They had to be kidding.

I remember the sheer terror at the thought of sticking that needle into my skin. I remember how ridiculously long and sharp that needle looked to me. I remember the juice pouring out of the orange as I stabbed it over and over with that syringe. I could not believe that this was really happening. I just kept closing my eyes, hoping that when I opened them I would be tucked warm and cozy in my own bed laughing at how crazy this dream had been. When I opened my eyes, however, I was still in the hospital. I was really sitting on the edge of this hospital bed with a syringe in one hand and an orange in the other. I was really living an absolute nightmare.

That day I heard the word "insulin" for the very first time. "Insulin" was, the doctor explained, the medication that would, in essence, keep me alive from here on out. It was the medication that I could no longer live without. Insulin was the stuff that was normally made in my pancreas (whatever that was) but that now I had to inject into my body because my pancreas did not work anymore. Up until that very day, I did not even know that I had a pancreas, much less that it could stop working if I ate too many Hershey's kisses. My nine year old mind blamed this entire disease on the Hershey's kisses. I was way too immature to understand what was really happening in my body and way too shocked by all of this new information to really care. I did not want to understand: I just wanted it all to go away.

This nightmare that had become my life was scarier than anything that I could have dreamed up in my own imagination. I was nine years old, I was sitting in a hospital, and I had just been diagnosed with type 1 diabetes. In one hand I held an orange, in the other hand I held a syringe with a very large, very sharp needle, and I had tears running down both of my cheeks. I was absolutely terrified. I imagine most nine year olds would have been terrified at this point as well. I was a very young child – I did not know about diseases like I do now. In my mind the world was free: free from disease, free from drugs, free from needles, and free to eat whatever one craved. Free, that is, until that moment. This loss of freedom from disease and drugs and needles and diet devastated me. Never before had I ever considered being "diseased." Never before had I considered that I might have to cause myself pain in order to survive. Never before had I considered that I might have to give myself an injection – much less more than one. Never before had I considered that I might have to be dependent on some type of drug in order to survive. Never before had I imagined that a sickness could exist that did not have a cure – and that I would be stricken with it. Never before had I considered that I might have to face one of my biggest fears: needles.

Along with my biggest fear came the biggest challenge in my life since the Ford Punt, Pass, and Kick Competition. This challenge was taking my first injection. Back then, the needles were much larger than they are today. Thank God for technology – the needles have become much smaller over the years. However, technology could not change that moment in time. As I sat on the edge of my hospital bed, the nurse was instructing me that this needle I had in my hand had to go into my thigh. I was shaking nervously. I was crying. I was absolutely terrified. Yet I was trying as hard as I could to be brave. I did not want anyone else to have to give me my injections – especially my mother. My mother was a nurse, but a boy does reach an age where he does not want to have to depend on his mother all the time. I was definitely at that age; and, I did not want anyone to feel sorry for me. I wanted to be strong. I wanted to brave. I wanted to make my parents proud of me. I wanted these nurses to stop patting my back like I was a little baby. So, I told myself that I was going to put this needle in my leg, even if it was the last thing I ever did. I told myself that I was going to put this needle in my leg, even though I was completely terrified to do it. The nurse held my hand to guide me. I was crying to hard that I could not even see the needle or my leg. As I cried I told that nurse that I was ready to face my fear. I just kept shouting "Okay!!" as that nurse held my hand and counted down slowly from three to one. Once I heard her finally get to down to "one," I looked through my tears and cried out in pain as that nurse forced me to shove that needle into my thigh. I thought I was going to die.

I can still visualize that needle poking out of my leg. It was almost surreal. It has been thirty-seven years since I first shoved that needle into my thigh, and it feels like it was only yesterday. The visual is still quite clear in my mind. It took all of the strength and all of the bravery I had to get that needle into my leg, but I did it. I did it through the fear and through the tears and through the pain. I did it. After I shoved that needle into my thigh for the very first time, I then pushed insulin into my body for the very first time. I still remember what the insulin felt like entering my body. The insulin was very calming. I remember the feeling of knowing that this was the "life source" for my new body. I then remember the relief of finally being able to remove that needle from my thigh. When that first injection was over, I fell back onto my hospital bed and cried tears of relief, sadness, and of the realization that this was just the first injection of many to come.

As I laid there in that hospital bed staring at the ceiling, I still remember wondering why that day had to happen, and why it had to happen that way. I was still hoping that this was all just a horrible nightmare, a simple bad dream, and that I would wake up any minute in my bed wondering how in the world my imagination had invented such a crazy dream. But it was not a dream. This day was really happening. I was quick to realize that I had to get used to every day happening like this one. I had to get used to doctors. I had to get used to giving myself injections. I had to get used to the "new Gregg" that I had woken up to today: the "new Gregg" with diabetes.

The "new Gregg" was somewhat different than the "old Gregg." The "new Gregg" had gotten much thinner than the "old Gregg" during hospitalization. I went from being the huskiest kid in my class to being the skinniest. The "old Gregg" was my dream. The "old Gregg" was in fourth grade, yet had the skill and the size to play on the sixth grade football team. I was so proud of the "old Gregg." He was popular. He was humorous. He could take out guys twice his size on the football field. I decided that I was going to do everything I could to keep as much of the "old Gregg" alive as possible.

Although I did not realize this at first, I was in the hospital for quite some time. I was quite shocked to learn that I had been in my Hershey kiss-induced coma for eight days. Once I awoke from my coma, I was kept in the hospital for a few weeks longer so that the doctors and nurses could keep an eye on my blood glucose levels and teach me how to recognize when my body needed insulin or glucose. While I was there, I lost about twenty pounds. I had hyperglycemic moments and hypoglycemic moments. I found entertainment while I was in the hospital in going from room to room to make people laugh.

That was the "old Gregg" coming alive in the "new Gregg" that had diabetes. My mother and father did everything they could to keep my spirits up and to help me accept that I had diabetes. I thank them for that. They still treated me like the child I was even though this disease had dropped the responsibility of an adult in my lap. When they were with me, I felt normal. My mother and father were there as much as they could be and they did not treat me any differently. The nurses at the hospital, I have to admit, spoiled me. It did not take me very long to figure out that I could drop a few tears and a nurse would come running. They were truly wonderful. The nurses helped me with my injections, but encouraged me to give them to myself as much as possible. Despite all of their efforts, I never really got used to taking the injections while I was in the hospital. I cried every single time and had to literally be forced to give myself that injection every single time. But none of that really mattered – the injections had to be taken. Just like my blood glucose levels had to be taken. Back then there was no such thing as a glucose meter or blood tester. Back then there were only small sticks that tested my urine for excess sugar. I had to be trained to use these sticks, read the results on the sticks, and to try and recognize my body's signals of hyperglycemia and hypoglycemia.

This was a whole new world. I took on this new world like any nine year old boy would – praying it would go away and leaning totally on my parents.

I remember leaving the hospital as the "new Gregg." Although I had diabetes, I convinced myself that life was not going to be any different. I was going to be normal and be the same person that I had been all along. I was going to be just like the "old Gregg." It wasn't too long after the "new Gregg" arrived home from the hospital, though, that I realized life WAS going to be different. I realized that I was going to have to accept the "new Gregg" whether I wanted to or not.

I still remember the first hypoglycemic reaction that I had after I came home from the hospital. I remember feeling so hungry and so dizzy and so shaky that it frightened me. I remembered feeling the same way a few times in the hospital, but this time there were no nurses here to help me. I remembered that when I felt like this, the nurses had always brought me something sweet to eat or drink. Looking back, I was probably given glucose drinks, but to my nine year old mind they were just something sweet to drink. With this in mind, I went to the kitchen to find something sweet so that I could make this feeling go away. What I found was a bag of Tootsie pops. (Hershey's kisses had become banned from our home.) As I ate them one after another, I remember thinking that this was actually great! My nausea and dizziness were going away, and it was all thanks to Tootsie pops!! I thought the doctors were all wrong – I thought I NEEDED all this SUGAR in order to make it! The sugar was actually making me feel BETTER! Better, that is, until my mom found me in the kitchen surrounded my wrappers and empty lollipop sticks. It was then that my mom gave me the bad news: she told me that I ate too much sugar and now I had to have an injection of insulin. That one little word – insulin - completely burst my bubble. My happy moment was destroyed in a matter of seconds. When my mom brought me the syringe, I began to cry. How could Tootsie pops do this to me? It just was not fair! It was not fair that I now had to have the dreaded insulin injection after just enjoying some candy. I now had caused myself to need that dreaded insulin injection by eating too much sugar. I absolutely could not believe it.

Now that I was home from the hospital, it was time to go back to school. I absolutely dreaded it. I dreaded having to be in school everyday and face this disease on my own. I wanted my mother and father to be there to help me, but that was impossible. I remember crying to my father. I remember not wanting to go back to school. I did not want to face my friends as the "new Gregg" with diabetes. I was not the "old Gregg" anymore and I was afraid. I was weak now. I was skinny now. I was diseased now. I was different now. I was afraid of what everyone would think of me. My spirit was fragile, and now, so was my body.

It was now time for me to face life as the "new Gregg." It was time for me to grow up. I was now going to grow up the "new Gregg" with diabetes. I could not imagine how my life was going to change, but I was ready. I was ready to return to what I hoped would be as close to a normal life and normal childhood as possible. I was returning to school and growing up.

Chapter Two

Growing Up with Diabetes

The day I that returned to school was "Presidential Fitness Day." This particular day had always been a favorite of mine. "Presidential Fitness Day" was the day when the school held a competition. This competition involved physical fitness: who could perform the most push-ups, pull-ups, sit-ups, run the farthest, and so on. The "old Gregg" had been known as one of the strongest kids in the school, and had always done extremely well in the competition. "Presidential Fitness Day" had always been MY day. It had always been my day to be on top of the world. It had always been my day to win. It had always been my day to be the junior-varsity football player that always came out on top. The "old Gregg" was the champion on this day. The "new Gregg" did not do so well. The "new Gregg" was not a champion. My first day back at school as the "new Gregg" was horrible. I failed miserably. I was no longer one of the strongest kids in school: I was now one of the weakest kids in school. I could not even do one pull-up. After five push-ups I felt like I was going to pass out. I could not do anything that I used to do. I was weak. However, this weakness gave me a new determination: I became determined to get my strength back. I became determined to overcome this disease. I became determined to become normal again. I became determined to become the "old Gregg" again.

Although I had changed physically, mentally I was still the same "old Gregg." All of my friends were very supportive, and they treated me just the same as before I got diabetes. Most of them even forgot about it after a while since I looked normal. I do not really think that they understood all of the dynamics of my disease, but they liked it when I shared the candy that I was now allowed to keep in my pocket. I made it back onto the football team, and managed to make the rest of elementary school seem somewhat normal. I merged into the lifestyle of a child with diabetes – injections included – with pride and strength. I exercised everyday. I pushed hard to be normal. I became stronger everyday. I made the wrestling team. I continued on with football. I took insulin injections in the bathroom, and sometimes had to manage hypoglycemic attacks in class, without anyone really seeming to notice. Even my teachers seemed not to notice my disease, even though I had hoped they would be some form of help. Everyone knew that I had to take injections now and carry candy in my pocket, but no one really seemed to care why. No one wanted to know why, and no one wanted to help. I was forced to face this disease on my own. And I was doing it successfully.

As we moved on as a family, and I moved on with my new life, we headed to a new town: Phoenix, Arizona. As we traveled, my dad had big promises of swimming pools, big fun, and of me living my dreams. It was wonderful to move to a new town where no one knew I had diabetes. Even though I was skinny now, no one knew that I used to be bigger and stronger.

Of course, my new school had a bully. And, of course, this bully made me a target. But, I will leave that story out. My real fight was the fight with diabetes. To me, diabetes was a lot worse than a bloody nose.

Since I was in a new town – I had left all of my friends and the hospital behind in Flagstaff – I managed to keep my diabetes a secret. I hid the fact that I had a disease very well. I seemed to function just like everybody else. I played hard and goofed off just like all of my new friends and just as I had before I got diabetes. I had to drink a little extra water, but no one really seemed to notice. I took my insulin injections in the bathroom so no one would see me. If I felt like my blood sugar was dropping, I just snuck a piece of candy into my mouth and went on like everything was just fine. I functioned just like all of the other kids. No one knew that I had a disease at all – until I went into a COMA.

I do not remember entering the coma, but I remember waking up with the same fuzziness that I felt the first time I woke up from a diabetic coma. When I woke up, I looked around and realized that I was in the hospital. Once I realized where I was, the first thing I thought of was those sweet drinks they had given me in the hospital before. I was ready to get up and find a nurse to help me out. Before I got up, however, I looked down at my arms to see why they felt so sore. I was shocked to see that my arms were black and blue. I had IV's sticking into my arms: IV's that had obviously been there for quite some time. I only had one IV last time I was in the hospital. All of these needles poking into my arms was completely new for me. From what I was told, I had been in a coma. I had been in a coma for four days. This coma was caused by – of course- some complication with my diabetes. I was told this was very common. Without the blood testers, insulin pumps, and wonderful advancements we have today, controlling blood glucose levels was a completely different ball game. My mother told me I should thank God that I survived this hypoglycemic attack. She was crying again. I recall asking my mother why this kept happening to me and why no one could make me any better. She said that doctors were "trying" but that so far no one knew how to make me any better. I used to have these visions of chemists in their labs wearing their white coats and mixing different colored liquids in an endless quest to find a cure for my disease. I had a hard time understanding how doctors could know so much about my disease, but not enough to cure it. I began to realize that my life would never be normal again. I began to realize that diabetes had much more control of my life than I did. I began to realize, even as a child, that if doctors could not make me better, no one could.

For the second time in my short life, I left the hospital and returned to school. For the second time in my life I returned to school as the skinny "new Gregg." I remember that I was as skinny as a rail – there were not even muscles on my body. When I looked in the mirror, I felt like there was nothing but a skeleton staring back at me. At least the children at the new school had never seen the "old Gregg." As the "new Gregg," I tried to fit in with the other boys. I tried to do everything that all of the other boys did. It had not been as difficult to keep up with the other boys before my coma as it was now. Even though I was weak and tired, I really tried to be just like everyone else. With this new disease I suddenly felt like the "ugly duckling." I felt like no matter how hard that I tried, I would never be normal. I felt like I was always going to be "diabetic".

Outside of my school, there was a large electrical box. Everyone has seen them: the large green or beige metal boxes that protect all the wires running into the schools. This particular box was green, and was about four feet tall. All of the boys in my class would push themselves up onto the top of this electrical box and hang out. Once I made some friends I was invited to hang out on this box with the other boys. I remember like it was just yesterday the first time that I tried to push myself up onto this box and hang out, too. I could not do it. I tried several times, but failed every single time. My body had not fully recovered from the coma, and I just did not have the strength to get up onto that box. I was so embarrassed. I felt so weak. The other boys made fun of me – calling me a "wimp" and other choice words. They were all laughing at me. None of them understood that I had a disease. They just saw me as a skinny little wimp. None of them understood that I wanted to be normal. None of them understood that I wanted to be strong – just strong enough to be normal. None of them understood that they were kicking me when I was already down.

After I shared this experience with him through teary eyes, my father decided to buy me a weight set so that I could build my strength back up. This weight set was wonderful – complete with a bench and plenty of free weights. Before I knew it, I felt like I had found a way to beat diabetes! I thought that lifting weights would make me normal. And it almost did. Weight-lifting strengthened me so much. It gave me a chest. It gave me arms. It gave me good posture. It gave me better health. It gave me strength – the strength that I craved so much. I was finally gaining enough strength to be normal. Lifting weights gave me confidence – confidence I had lost with my diagnosis. I was finally becoming the "old Gregg" again.

With this confidence came new opportunities. One of these opportunities was karate. Once I had joined karate, I remember punching and kicking everywhere I went. Just like most boys at that time, I idolized Bruce Lee. I even tore my corduroy pants trying to kick like Bruce Lee! (Yes, I wore corduroy pants!) Karate was not my only new opportunity at that time. Once I got my strength up and began to have fewer and fewer blood glucose related problems, my parents allowed me to have a paper route. I loved my paper route. My paper route gave me confidence. My paper route gave me a paycheck. My paper route gave me freedom – freedom to buy all the sugar I wanted!!!

Right around the corner from my house was a little store called *The Village Market*. *The Village Market* became a gold mine for me. I was a kid with a pocket full of money and a craving: a craving for sweets. It was only a short amount of time, maybe a few weeks, before my parents found out that I was buying a large amount of sweets at *The Village Market*. I remember once in particular, before my parents caught on to my game, when I bought a chocolate cream pie. Yes, I bought an entire chocolate cream pie. I still remember just how delicious that pie was. I think that it tasted even better because I knew that I was not supposed to have it. After I bought that pie, I went to the playground just down the street to hide. This playground was my normal hiding place: the place where I would hide and eat the sweets that I would buy. This playground had one of those big concrete tunnels right in the middle. I bought that chocolate cream pie and ran as fast as I could into the middle of that concrete tunnel.

Anyone that saw me probably thought that I was a thief on the run because I held that pie to my chest and ran as fast as I could. I hid in that tunnel, looked out each side of the tunnel to be sure that the coast was clear, and ate the whole thing with my hands. It tasted like a dream come true. I licked every single drop of off of my fingers. I felt great. I was completely satisfied with myself. Well, I was satisfied until, of course, I began to feel the effects of hyperglycemia. I began to realize that I had just caused myself, again, to need insulin. Again, that dreaded injection.

Since I had been in a coma, my friends now knew that I had diabetes. They did not really know what that meant and I did not really know how to explain it so that they would understand. All my friends really understood was that I loved to eat sweets and I had to have an injection from time to time. Back then, I could make it most days with just one injection. One really big injection. I only had to have more than one injection if I went crazy with the sweets. I think it was the exercise. I would run around non-stop – just like every other kid I knew. The only difference between me and the other kids was the diabetes. I remember beginning to recognize when my blood glucose level was dropping, and then eating so many sweets I would almost get sick. At that time I did not have the rebound effects that I have now if I indulge too much after hypoglycemia, unless of course I went out of control (like with the chocolate cream pie). The effects of all the exercise I was getting were on my side. I swam. I played baseball with my friends. I took karate. I had a paper route. I lifted my weights everyday. I did my best to be as normal as possible and have as much fun as possible. I had nothing but fun, until, of course, I began to enter my teenage years.

Entering my teenage years with diabetes was a new challenge. Not only was I struggling with diabetes; as soon as I began my teenage years, my parents divorced. That was extremely difficult for me. My father had been so good to me. My father was the one who took care of me when I had my reactions, he held me when I cried, he encouraged me when I felt weak, he had bought me the weight set to build my strength, and then he was gone. Not only did I have to live with diabetes, I now had to live with diabetes without my father. I missed his support more than I had ever missed anything. But, life went on and so did I.

As a result of the divorce, my mother, my brother, and I moved again. Again I was entering a new school, and again I had the chance

36

to hide my diabetes. Well, I suppose I did not hide it as much as I just did not mention it unless it was absolutely necessary. I was still somewhat ashamed of my diabetes. I did not like having to explain it to everyone. Just like before, I would hide in the bathroom if I had to take an insulin injection, and slip some candy if I began to feel dizzy. I dealt with my diabetes as best as I could without the support of my father. I dealt with it like I dealt with going to the bathroom: sometimes it was inconvenient, but I had to do it anyway.

High school was again, a new challenge. One major challenge that I remember was playing on the basketball team. As part of our daily practice, the players on the team ran two miles. Since I did not want to be treated any differently or to have to explain my disease, I would always run just like everyone else – without stopping. On quite a few occasions I recall that I would barely make it back to the gymnasium. I would arrive back at the gym with such severe hypoglycemia that I would have to slam as many sodas as quickly as I could in order to prevent passing out. I told my coach that I had diabetes, but he did not understand diabetes and he did not really care to learn about it. He did not understand why I had to drink soda instead of water after a two mile run and, again, he did not really care why. The only thing he understood was that it took me a long time to get to the court for practice after the run, and he gave me a hard time about it. Again, I was dealing with this disease on my own. I felt like no matter how hard I tried to explain my disease, no one understood. And even worse was the fact that no one, not even my coach, really cared. The battle was all mine. I won the battle this time: I made it through the entire season without ending up in another coma.

At the end of the school year, we moved again. Again I was given the wonderful gift of a new school and new friends that had no idea that I had a disease. I spent half a year at that school – and no one ever knew I had diabetes.

Finally, I ended up at the high school where I would graduate. I played on the tennis team. I made friends in the neighborhood. I continued to lift weights. And it was at this time in my life that I also began to read bodybuilding magazines. As I read them, I began to realize that these magazines contained a plethora of knowledge: knowledge about "glycogen" or sugar. I also began to learn about chromium picolinate from these magazines. Chromium picolinate is something that helps insulin get into muscle cells, or enhances the effects of insulin. I was learning some wonderful things about supplements that were sold to make muscles bigger – but also had the added effect of regulating blood glucose levels. For the first time since my diagnosis I began to truly learn what insulin was really doing in my body. I began to stay on the cutting edge of nutrition information. I kept reading these magazines in order to learn how to build my muscles and regulate my blood glucose levels. These magazines were a blessing from God! I was getting bigger, I was getting stronger, and I was having fewer and fewer glycemic reactions. God had finally given me the knowledge I needed to stay healthy! Not to mention that these magazines were FULL of pictures of beautiful fitness models…

With bodybuilding aside, the high school years were definitely challenging for me, just like they were for everyone else. My body chemistry was changing, my hormones were going crazy, and my diabetes was on my mind most of the time. And, although I made everyone laugh, I was actually a little bit shy. I dealt with my shyness through comedy. I found unique ways to deal with all the challenges of high school – especially my disease. One way I dealt with my diabetes was, as usual, to hide it. I would pretend like it did not exist. Although I would pretend that I was just normal, I began to realize that

I had to use this time in my life to find a way to deal with my diabetes. Was I going to control my diabetes, or was it going to control me?

Again, as I went through the young years of my life, I did not have blood glucose monitors, insulin pumps, blood testers, or any of the major technologies that we have today. The only way that I had to deal with my diabetes was to take a large injection of insulin, eat lots of nutritious food, and exercise. I played tennis in high school, and managed to make it through the entire season without telling the coach that I had diabetes. I did not want to be treated any differently than anyone else. I did a good job of managing my blood glucose levels, so that my coaches and most of my friends did not have to know that I had a disease. It only became difficult when I became hypoglycemic. The main thing that is important is that I was finally managing my disease, and managing it well enough that no one knew that I was not normal.

As my body was changing my junior and senior year, I went through episodes of little to no energy that I now recognize as hyperglycemia. Hyperglycemia (high blood glucose levels) can be just as dangerous as hypoglycemia (low blood glucose levels). I began to realize when I was experiencing hyperglycemia just by my inability to focus mentally. When hyperglycemic attacks were extreme, I could not function physically, either. I dealt with this as best as I could – taking insulin in secrecy and always having a pocket full of candy just in case I took too much insulin during one of these attacks.

Although I began to have many more hyperglycemic attacks at this stage of my life, I was still able to do most of the things that I wanted to do. I worked construction in the summers and played sports during the school year. When I began to work construction, however, I began to have the hardest time with my blood glucose levels. In the summertime, I would get up at 4:00 o'clock in the morning and ride my bicycle to work. I would enter the construction site and begin mixing concrete at 5:00 o'clock. I had a hard time keeping up with these seasoned block layers in the heat, but somehow I managed to do it. Once the heat of the day kicked in, I would have numerous hypoglycemic reactions that would absolutely embarrass me. My boss seemed to get frustrated every time that I had to stop working and eat. Although I tried to explain it to him, my boss just did not understand my disease – he just thought I was a "growing boy." I did not want to have to battle this disease while working alongside these strong, grown men. But, sometimes, my body would just not do what I wanted it to do and the diabetes would take control of me. Despite embarrassing myself by eating constantly, I worked as hard as I could and earned respect on the job.

I went through so many different things growing up with diabetes. There are so many different emotions that go along with this disease. As I started to get into my middle teens and twenties, I mistakenly began to base my self-image on how people treated me when they found out that I had a disease. Of course, even without a disease the opinions of others can have a direct effect on your self-esteem at these ages. But, as I dealt with this disease, unsuccessfully hiding it from the world and being treated like I had a disease, I changed completely.

Most of the feelings that I had toward myself in my late teens and early twenties were, again, based on the way that others treated me at the time. I specifically remember that one of my doctors was so condescending to me that it was hurtful to keep my appointments. He was very unforgiving if my blood glucose levels were even a tiny bit off, even though I was just a child. He would tell me that if I did not learn to take care of this disease like an adult that I would die at a young age. Even as a teenager I was brought to tears by the statement this doctor made, and my mother was always angry with me when we left. She would spend the entire drive home preaching to me how important it was that I put my diabetes first and stop acting like a *child*. (They all seemed to forget that *I was still a child*.) I also recall that people could be very unkind once they found out that I had a disease. Diabetes was not as common as it is now, and no one really tried to understand it. Unfortunately, feelings began to arise in me that followed me around for quite a few years. I had feelings of guilt, of not being "good enough", of being "diseased". Every time that I heard someone mention to my mother that they were "so sorry" that her son had diabetes it hit me a little harder. I just wanted to be normal and to be seen as normal. I just wanted this disease to go away. But, of course, it did not.

I recall a specific incident in my early twenties when one of my friends was diagnosed with diabetes. I was working part time as security at a night club and was in some of the best shape of my life. A friend of mine came in quite often to see me, and on this one particular night he seemed very depressed. I asked my friend what had happened and he let me know that he had just been diagnosed with diabetes. What? I thought to myself. Did this guy just tell me that he has just been diagnosed with my disease? He was just as healthy looking as I was and he had no idea that I had the disease. I asked why he was so depressed about this, and he said to me that he was afraid. He said that he was afraid he was going to die. He said that he was afraid to take injections. He had the strength to say everything that I was feeling inside yet had been afraid to share all of these years. And when I told them that I had been diagnosed with diabetes as a young boy and would be more than willing to help him and be there for him, I though that he would cry. For the very first time since I was diagnosed with this disease I was the strong one. I was now the person that someone else with this disease was looking to for answers. I was a testimony. I was the guide. I was not diseased in the eyes of my friend: I was his savior.

The complexity of this disease is just way too much for some people. It is so much easier to just forget about this disease rather than to learn about it. It is difficult sometimes to know that this problem exists in my endocrine system, even though I look just fine. I like to refer to it as the "invisible killer". I wanted to be like the rest of the world. I wanted to just forget about my diabetes and hope that it would just go away. I wanted to forget how people treated me

44

differently when they found out that I had a disease. I wanted to forget what all the doctors were telling me: I would probably die from this disease and/or complications from it before I would even reach my forties. I wanted to forget that I had to have health insurance in order to be able to afford to survive. I wanted to forget that everyday I had to make a conscious effort to take care of myself. I wanted to go just one day as the "old Gregg" and not have to have that injection. I wanted to go back to that day when I ate those two bags of Hershey's kisses and make that day never happen. I wanted to forget about my blood glucose levels for just one day. Just one day.

Even after my diagnosis I had wonderful aspirations for my life. First I wanted to be a comedian. I enrolled in community college, but once I was enrolled I decided that I wanted to be a deejay. College with diabetes was not as difficult as high school had been. I had a good routine down where I would take my insulin before class and make it through the entire lecture without anyone knowing that I had a problem. It was also while in college that I decided to make good use of the gym and become a body builder. Ever since I had been diagnosed with diabetes I had been skinny. There was a time in high school where I had gained some weight, but a coma had taken all of that away. I saw college as my opportunity to become muscular. It did not take me very long to figure out that I could triple my dosage of insulin, pile on the calories, and then hit the gym to build muscles. Once I figured this out, I began to gain muscle. I began, at first, to gain the body of a normal man. Then, I began to gain LOTS of muscle. People began to look at me in a different way. People did not look at me like I had a disease – people looked at me like I had a great physique. When I did tell people I had diabetes, they could not believe that I had gained the muscle size that I had gained while having this disease. Most people had the idea that if someone had diabetes then they were also overweight. I was not overweight. I was muscular AND I was diabetic.

Since being muscular gave me such high self-esteem. I began to read every nutritional article that I could in order to change my body into a muscle machine. I remembered what I had learned from these magazines in high school and just added to the knowledge. I no longer desired to be a comedian, I no longer desired to be a deejay; I wanted to be a bodybuilder. I worked hard in school to become educated in nutrition and exercise. I realized that although I will have diabetes for the rest of my life, I could finally take on the challenge of having this disease and becoming more. I began to realize that it was a much bigger challenge for me to sit though a class, allowing my blood glucose levels to go sky high, than it was to exercise and make my body healthy. I finally realized that the worst thing I could do for my disease was sit still. I could not just sit and work my mouth and gluteus, so to speak. By exercising and following a healthy diet I became in such good control of my diabetes that, at the time, I forgot that I even had the disease. I could not believe that it took me over ten years to realize that control of this disease comes from exercise and nutrition. I want everyone with this disease to control it as I have. I want everyone with this disease to get excited about taking care of their body, so that it does not take care of them.

I finally had a successful routine. I woke up in the morning, drank a protein shake, took my insulin, and exercised. Also at this time (somewhere in my twenties) I was finally able to recognize my body signals – moodiness, indecisiveness, confusion, nausea - of hyperglycemia and hypoglycemia. I finally felt good. My body looked great, I felt fantastic, and I had my diabetes under control. Although I had diabetes, God had blessed me with the knowledge to control it.

As I look back, the strongest feelings that I had regarding my disease while growing up were feelings of guilt. I felt like I had done something wrong that caused me to get this disease. I even blamed the Hershey's kisses for the first few years. I felt like God was punishing me for something that I had done wrong. I felt like I was much more of a burden on my parents than my brother (who was normal) was. Those are probably the feelings that many of you with diabetes reading this book have. Guilt, embarrassment, shame – all of the feelings associated with being "different" or "diseased". I had to overcome those feelings in order to accept my disease. I had (and still do have) to tell myself that "I have", "I can", and "I will" overcome this disease. I have to constantly remind myself that I am blessed by God and will defeat this disease. We all are and we all will.

These feelings are the most difficult to overcome as a child. The best way to overcome these feelings is with support: support from family, friends, doctors, and occasionally outside sources. One of the best ways for me to face this disease was to surround myself with others that were just like me. I had the privilege one summer to spend a few weeks with children just like me that were suffering from this disease just like I was. I had the privilege to attend Diabetic Camp.

That summer gave me a renewed view of my disease and a new hope.

Chapter Three

Diabetic Camp

Diabetic camp was a wonderful time for me. Being surrounded by other children with my disease – children just like me – was very therapeutic. I went to camp in a beautiful area – Prescott, Arizona. I stayed in a beautiful cabin. There was horseback riding with a mini rodeo, barrel racing, hiking, swimming, and all of the outdoor activities that a child loves. There were doctors, nurses, and counselors. All of these people were fantastic people. These people gave their time and love to all of us children with diabetes. There were older men and women with diabetes, also, that helped us with everything. I remember, specifically, a man named Drew. Drew was a former professional football player. He was older, he was healthy, and he was in fantastic shape. You would never even know that he had diabetes unless he told you. He was very kind and understanding, and he, among others, made a positive impact on my life.

Camp was a wonderful place for a diabetic child to be outdoors. We learned how to set up camp; we learned how to fish, we swam, we learned how to start a campfire, we learned how to just be normal kids despite our disease. We even had a little dance at the end of camp. Of course, I was a stud back then and had numerous little ladies that wanted to be my date…but we won't talk about that. It was definitely therapeutic to feel free and normal with this disease. Camp provided me an outlet – I felt normal for the entire summer. It was fantastic.

I remember one doctor in particular who would make us laugh constantly. He was a doctor, but he also suffered from type 1 diabetes just like the rest of us. I remember how he would take his insulin injections through his t-shirt and never wince. My mother was not happy when I came home from camp doing the same thing…but we had quite a bit of fun with him. I recall how he would laugh when my friends and I would try and fool him on our blood glucose tests. We all had mouthwash that was a yellow color, and we would fill our urine test cups with that mouthwash instead of urine. Of course, no one was really fooled, but the doctors and nurses did laugh about it and encourage our humor and our youthfulness.

The reality that we had diabetes was never too far from our minds despite all of the fun. I remember one fellow camper had a severe hypoglycemic reaction while swimming and was found at the bottom of the swimming pool. Thank God we were surrounded by attentive doctors and nurses – he survived. It was a reminder to all of us, however, to remain vigilant when it comes to our disease. It made me much more aware of my body's hypoglycemic and hyperglycemic reactions so that the same thing would not happen to me.

As a whole, the most freedom that I ever felt as a child with diabetes was at camp. I was surrounded by children that were just like me and I was surrounded by people that knew how to take care of me. It is not like that in normal society. In normal society, no one really knows what is wrong with you or that you even have a disease. And if I have any type of glycemic reaction in normal society, no one really knows how to help. It was not like that at camp. At camp, everyone had snacks in their pocket just in case my blood glucose level, or anyone's blood glucose level, was dropping. The meals were amazing – great to eat and healthy for us, too. I felt so energetic everyday because I had the proper nutrition. I was taken such good care of that I will never forget it.

I personally recommend diabetic camp for any child that has diabetes. It will make such a positive difference in their lives to be surrounded by other children that have the same disease, the same fears, and the same desire to be understood. Every child with diabetes deserves this chance. Diabetic camp helped me learn to take care of myself and it also gave my parents a much needed break from the constant worry of my health. When I got home from camp, my parents and I were both refreshed and ready to tackle everyday life with diabetes with new energy. I had the time of my life at diabetic camp, and I would again recommend it to any child with diabetes. Check with the Americans with Diabetes Association at www.diabetes.org for more information.

Once I returned home from diabetic camp, I was ready to face my disease with a new hope and a new strength. I was getting close to the age of moving out of my parents home and moving on with my life as an adult. I finally realized that I could face this disease on my own and that I was not the only one that suffered from this disease. I finally realized that I could make it on my own.

Chapter Four

On My Own With Diabetes

Diabetes has now become a major part of my life. I experienced the major part of my childhood with it and, unless a cure is found, I will die with it. (But not **of** it). Once I left home I did not have the parental guidance that I had before in dealing with my disease, but I grew up and moved on just like any other normal human being. I took life head on – gaining as much knowledge as I could and taking as good of care of my body as possible. I listened to my doctors and again gained large amounts of knowledge from bodybuilding magazines. Once I moved out on my own, the hardest part of diabetes was the cost. I had a job, but I struggled to pay rent just like everyone in their twenties. Thank God I had qualified for state health insurance to help ease the cost of having diabetes. When I had extra money, it went to pharmacies and doctors instead of to partying and going out like with most of my friends. As a child, I had never considered, just like everyone else on earth, what life would be like on my own. I had never considered that I would have to make sure that I had health insurance just to be able to afford survival. At first, my Mom had kept me on her insurance plan, but later helped me sign up through the state once I was able to qualify. It was not the best in the world, but I was able to see my doctor and afford my insulin, and that is what was important.

Being out in the workforce brought a whole new light to my disease. It did not take my employers long to notice that I was not "normal." It also did not take them long to notice that I was taking injections and eating candy. Thankfully, I was over my reluctance to let others know that I have diabetes. The nice thing about being an adult was that I was rarely treated any differently once I shared the fact that I have diabetes. I was still expected to do my job, and although my employers knew that I had diabetes, they did not know much about it and did not really seem to care. I was finally treated like everyone else and I was thankful for that.

Through most of my younger years, there was no such thing as a blood glucose monitor. I spent most of my life just "winging it" as far as my blood glucose levels were concerned, and I was able to recognize whether I was hyperglycemic or hypoglycemic at any given time. Since I was exercising so much at the time, I was able to keep my blood glucose at mostly normal levels. Again, I used the knowledge that I had gained in my nutrition classes in college and from reading bodybuilding magazines. I followed the suggested high-protein diets and managed to mold my body into exactly what I wanted it to be – muscular.

Once I reached the fine age of twenty-one, I began to want to go to bars and drink beer with my friends. With my disease, one of the worst things I could do is drink alcohol. Alcohol has quite the yo-yo effect on blood glucose levels and it is not the wisest choice of beverages for someone with diabetes. Despite this fact, I was a twenty-one year old man and I was going to do whatever I wanted. Although I continued to stay active, I began to have some trouble with hyperglycemia not long after my partying days began. I began to have difficulty waking up in the mornings – with what I thought was a hangover just like everyone else had. I was wrong. The alcohol was affecting my diabetes in such a way that was causing extreme hyperglycemia in the early morning hours. On nights that I did not consume alcohol, I began to notice how much better I felt in mornings and how much easier it was for me to get out of bed. Once blood glucose monitors were invented, I discovered that alcohol would cause me to wake up with extremely high blood glucose levels. But, since blood glucose monitors had not yet been invented at the time, I just went by how my body felt. I felt so much better and so much healthier when I did not drink alcohol, so I stopped. My diabetes had given me the gift of discipline with my diet, and this was no exception. It did not take me very long after I stopped consuming alcohol to get my blood glucose levels back under control and to start feeling normal again.

As an adult, I was able to handle hypoglycemic reactions much better than when I was a child. I did have a few "close calls", however. There was one incident at a local restaurant while I was dining with my friends that could have been deadly had I not been aware of my body signals. I was beginning to feel my body's tell-tale signs of hypoglycemia – dizziness, nausea, confusion, shakiness – and asked the waitress to please bring me a soda. Well, little did I know that everyone else at the table was drinking diet soda, so that was what I was brought, also. After I had downed about four of them, one of my close friends that knew about and understood my disease asked if I was alright. I told him that my blood glucose level was dropping and that soda normally brought it up, but I was still feeling low. That is when he asked me if diet soda had any sugar in it. As soon as he asked me that question, I realized that I was probably drinking diet soda and I immediately asked the waitress for regular soda. Thank God that I did. I could barely speak by the time she brought the regular soda to me, and my blood glucose level had dropped so low that I ended up drinking five sodas before I felt better. Although I was very full and very bloated, I was thankful that my friend knew about my disease and cared enough to help me out. I have learned from that experience: if I feel as if my blood glucose level is dropping in a restaurant, I make sure that I request "regular" soda.

Another "close call" with hypoglycemia occurred while I was camping with some friends. When I had packed my cooler, along with my insulin I had packed extra snacks (donuts, sweet candies, cookies) for myself just in case I had a hypoglycemic reaction. The particular people I was camping with did not know that I have diabetes. When I had gone to sleep that night, unbeknownst to me, the guys I was camping with had raided my cooler and had eaten everything in it. I woke up early in the morning, before everyone else, sweating and feeling extremely nauseous. I realized that I was having a hypoglycemic reaction, and went to my cooler for something sweet.

When I opened my cooler, the only thing in it was my insulin shot. At that point, I began to panic. I woke everyone up, explained to them the best that I could that I had a disease that required me to eat sugar in order to survive, and begged them rush me to the nearest store for food. Although they did not quite understand, they had seen the syringe in my cooler and understood that I had to be telling the truth. Thank God we were only about ten minutes from the nearest store. They threw me into the truck and got me the sugar that my body desperately needed. That experience taught me something: it taught me to protect myself. I realized that with diabetes you have to carry around some form of sugar, and that everyone wants to eat that sugar! I realized that I was better off making sure that I kept my sugar in my pocket so that it would still be there when I needed it rather than let anyone know that I was carrying around something sweet. It is amazing how those without diabetes think that they need sugar just as much as I do.

It was not long after this had occurred that I decided to move in with my father. I had not lived with my father since my early teens when he and my mother had divorced. I was a man now and my father and I were anxious to get to know each other again. I remember what great care he had taken of me when I was young and how he had always been particularly sensitive to the fact that I had diabetes. While I was living with him, my father signed me up for this program at the local hospital where I could see older men and women with diabetes and the long term toll that this disease had taken on their health. I was shocked at what I saw. Some of these people had failing kidneys, pancreatic cancer, amputated feet, and a large number of them were blind. Most of these people did not have very good nutrition, and it became very clear to me that nutrition was an important part of leading a normal life with diabetes. I remember one lady in particular, however, that I thought was in fantastic shape. She exercised, she lifted weights - and she was blind and her kidneys were failing. She had suffered from type 1 diabetes for almost 50 years and had not followed a very nutritious diet and had only recently begun to exercise. Her lack of knowledge about her disease had caused her life to become miserable. That is one woman that I will never forget. I will always remember the sadness behind her blind eyes. I will always remember her as a testament to good nutrition. As a diabetic, that woman made me realize that good nutrition could save my life. I will always thank my father for opening my eyes to how important it was and still is for me to take care of my body along with fighting my disease. He showed me that if I do not take care of my body – it will take care of me.

At the time, I also had a close friend named Scott. Scott was just like me – he had type 1 diabetes. He did not take as good of care of himself as I did: he had poor nutrition and he was a smoker. I hated cigarettes. Thankfully I could not stand the smell of them and had absolutely no desire to poison this beautiful body that I had built with exercise and good nutrition. Anyway, Scott and I became close due to our disease. We had met as young children at diabetic camp and remained close as adults. We spoke of glycemic reactions, the smell of insulin and hiding our disease. I also urged him to stop smoking and take better care of his body. I told him about the people I had observed at the hospital with my father and how our disease had taken such a terrible toll on most of their bodies. Scott did not heed the warning. He continued to smoke and follow a very unhealthy diet. I remember how shocked I was that someone could know how bad this disease can be if you do not take care of yourself and choose not to take of themselves anyway. I remember how shocked I was that this guy could run around, eat what he wanted, smoke cigarettes, have diabetes, and look perfectly healthy. I also remember how shocked I was when I got the phone call that he had died from complications with his diabetes when he looked just fine to me only days before. I am still shocked. I am still shocked that this disease can take your life so quickly, as it did his. I will always miss him, and I will also remember him as a testament to good nutrition as well. I do not want to be taken by this disease at a young age. Even at forty-five years old I am way too young to let this disease take my life. I am thankful to God that I have gained the knowledge of good nutrition and physical fitness that allow me to stay on top of this deadly disease. I want to be a LIVING testament to diabetes management – not a memorial.

After Scott passed away, I gained the desire to become more active in spreading diabetes awareness. It was at this time that I was given the opportunity to attend a "Diabetes Expo" that came to Phoenix, Arizona. While at the expo, I also had the opportunity to educate younger children with diabetes about the importance of good nutrition and physical fitness. At the expo I realized how normal diabetes actually looked. These children looked just like everyone else. They had the same hairstyles, the same clothes, the same attitude, but they also had diabetes. I came to realize that all of the silly things that I had worried about as a child were just that: silly things. No one could look at me and tell that I had this disease. I did not look different. I did not have this blinking sign on my forehead that read: *Caution: victim of diabetes.* Seeing these children was such a positive experience for me. I realized that they were dealing with this disease just as I had dealt with it. They dealt with it one day at a time and tried to have as normal a childhood as possible. They hide their disease from their friends, take insulin injections in the bathroom, sneak candy into their mouths when they feel hypoglycemic, and they pray for a cure everyday just like I did. I still pray for a cure everyday so that children in the future can have a normal life.

One of the most important lessons that anyone with diabetes can learn is to take care of themselves. Even if you are working a minimum wage job – washing dishes, bartending, bussing tables, pouring cement – all of those things that I did, it is important to do the best that you can do and take the very best care of your body. Most of the employers at these jobs treated me pretty well. I worked late hours and was able to sleep late. I loved to sleep late. Mornings were the hardest times for me – my blood glucose level was either way too high, which made me not want to get up, or way too low, which made me binge eat and want to go back to sleep. I enjoyed the jobs that allowed me to sleep as late as I wanted. Although these jobs were not the most glamorous, they did allow me the extra time I needed to go to the gym and exercise. I was still in excellent shape at the end of my twenties and as I entered my thirties. I was still reading the bodybuilding magazines and still experiencing large muscle gains with my manipulation of insulin. I had learned how to use my insulin to better benefit my body and experience large muscle growth. I slept late, went to the gym, rested again, and worked nights. For me, it was the ideal diabetes management program. I used what I had to my advantage. Then, I got the call for something better.

I had applied numerous times for different jobs within the City of Phoenix, Arizona. I wanted these jobs for two reasons: one reason was that most of the jobs paid extremely well and allowed for second shift hours so that I would not have to change my routine. The second reason was that the City of Phoenix had one of the best health insurance plans that a diabetic could imagine. My state insurance benefits were lessening every year and I needed steady employment that would provide better health insurance. Finally, I got a call from the Parks Department with the City of Phoenix. There was an opening for a Groundskeeper, complete with no benefits. Although the money was not great, the opportunity to have insurance in the future and possibly advance to higher levels within the Parks Department was enough to make me say yes. It was hard work at first. My supervisor at the time had me moving large boulders, due to my muscle size. I was under the impression that he was glad to have someone of my size and strength on staff. I did not tell my supervisor that I had diabetes, as I did not want to burst his bubble of excitement at having such a "strong young man" on staff. With this new job I did not feel diseased – I felt needed. I always kept snacks in my pocket and always took my insulin when my body needed it. I felt great. I still worked nights while I had this job, and the money was coming along nicely with two jobs. I finally made full time with the city, and my benefits kicked in. I was able to work only my city job and no longer had to work at night, and I now had the health insurance package that I had desperately needed. Although my schedule had to be turned completely around; I got up early, went to work, went to the gym, and then went to sleep, my body was now running like a well oiled machine. I was eating well and taking care of my body. Although the lack of health insurance when I first took the job had caused me to not see the doctor as often as I should have (my state insurance was cancelled because I made too much money when I began working for the city) I felt like I had my diabetes under the best control of my life. I looked phenomenal. I felt fantastic. I was the pride of my new employer. This was the life that I had always wanted. I was healthy and I was happy. THEN I WAS STRUCK WITH DISASTER.

One summer morning while I was working, I noticed this little black dot in the center of my visual field. I did not really think much of it at the time. I thought that maybe I had been looking up at the sun too long, or that maybe I was dehydrated and needed a break. By the middle of the day, however, this little black dot had turned into this little black "fish" swimming around in my visual field. It was there when I closed my left eye. It was there when I closed my right eye. No matter how many times that I blinked, it did not go away. By the end of the day, this little fish had turned into a big fish taking up most of my visual field. This was the most shocking thing that has ever happened to me. I mean, this ranks up there with being diagnosed with a deadly disease. Here I was, in my early thirties, in phenomenal shape, finally happy with the status of my life; and this huge darkness was overtaking my vision. This darkness was overtaking my vision like a black oil spill on a beautifully painted canvas. That evening when I went to bed I prayed that this darkness would be gone by morning. It wasn't. The next morning, I woke up, opened my eyes and expected everything to be back to normal. It wasn't. I called my supervisor and tried to explain what was happening to me. He advised me to skip work and go to the ophthalmologist. I heeded his advice. That is where it began. That is where I got the news that my entire life was going to change – again. By the time I got to the ophthalmologist, my vision was almost completely gone. I was afraid. I was afraid in a way that made me nauseous and filled my body with uncontrollable shakiness. I was afraid beyond sticking needles in my leg and keeping candy in my pocket. This fear was much more real to me. I thought that I was healthy. I took vitamins. I followed a nutritious diet. I exercised every single day. I thought that I had my diabetes under control. Then I got the news. This black hole in my vision was not a fluke. It was not going to go away. I not only had diabetes: I had Diabetic Retinopathy.

Chapter Five

Diabetic Retinopathy

Where will I go with my blindness?
What will I see?
Who will I recognize?
What does the future hold for me
When my eyes do not see?
I hold to your hand so tight, O Lord;
Wondering, thinking, imagining
Only what I used to see.
How will I ever have a family?
Why will it be
That I will raise someone I will never see?
I do not understand my pain;
I do not understand this defeat.
Is it over for me?
Am I a young man that will never see?
I do not know where I will go.
I do not know who will take care of me.
I do know that I am a man that must move on:
A man that cannot see.
I hold on tight to my dreams.
Though I know that the Lord makes my path for me:
Where will this path lead?
Where will I go with my blindness?
What will I see?

In all my time with this disease I had never really heard the

term "diabetic retinopathy." I did recall the blind lady at the hospital I

went to visit with my father quite a few years earlier, but I did not realize that she had gone blind directly from diabetes. No one had ever really explained to me that blindness could happen as a direct result of my disease or that it could happen this way. I had been warned that my kidneys could fail if I did not control my hyperglycemic reactions. I had been warned that I could lose my feet if I did not control my hypoglycemic reactions. I had even been warned that I could die in my sleep if my hypoglycemic reactions became severe while I was sleeping. But no one ever warned me that within twenty-four hours my vision could be almost completely gone due to this disease. Needless to say, I was a little shocked when I heard the diagnosis.

My ophthalmologist was Dr. Melvin Gerber. Dr. Gerber was an older gentleman, very nice, and very sympathetic. I recall that while I was lying there in his office chair, waiting for my pupils to dilate from the drops I was given, I could not believe what was happening. I had thought, especially at this point in my life, that I finally had my disease under control. I just could not believe that I was so strong, so young, and yet so strongly affected by my disease. I was very afraid: my palms were sweaty, my heart was pounding, and I was asking a million questions. I just wanted good news. I wanted to hear that this was just a fluke and that everything was going to be just fine. Dr. Gerber looked around in my eyes for what seemed like an eternity before he began to give me the news. The news that he gave to me was not the news that I had wanted to hear and it was not the news that I had prayed to hear.

Dr. Gerber informed me that I had a tear in the blood vessels in my vitreous fluid in my eye. The vitreous fluid, he explained, is the jelly-type fluid in the back of the eye. This fluid is full of blood vessels, and sometimes with diabetes these blood vessels tend to swell. Once these blood vessels swell, it is very easy for them to tear. Once they are torn, the blood vessels leak blood into the vitreous fluid. Once the blood is in the vitreous fluid, it just sits there and causes the "oil spill" that I was seeing. Dr. Gerber then explained to me that the bleeding had to be stopped immediately in order for the dark spots in my vision not to get any larger and further damage to my vision to be caused. He explained to me that he would be using a laser IMMEDIATELY in order to stop the bleeding in my eyes. I was overcome to say the least. Here was this doctor telling me that if I wanted to continue to have the gift of sight that I needed to have laser surgery immediately. And, of course, all of this was due to my diabetes. Without this disease, this never would have happened to me. I was devastated that once again my diabetes had taken some sort of tragic toll on my life. Once again, although I was only in my thirties, I was dealing with the serious effects that this devastating disease was having on my body..

I agreed to have the laser surgery that day. I remember that as I was getting ready for surgery, drops were put into my eyes and I was then to wait for them to dilate. As I was waiting, a television was turned on and I instantly heard Bob Barker hosting "The Price is Right". I remember laughing somewhat at the fact that this office had a television in the waiting room for people that could not see. I still chuckle at the thought; and I am thankful that at the time I had at least one reason to laugh. I suppose that the office staff had a sense of humor.

Once my eyes were dilated, Dr. Gerber performed the laser surgery. I cannot describe to you the amount of pain I felt as soon as that laser hit my eye. I remember gripping my chair as tight as I could and praying for the pain to stop. I had been warned that there would be some pain, but I had no idea that it would be of this magnitude. Thank God that the surgery only took about ten minutes. That was the longest ten minutes of my life thus far. The good news was that the "bleeders" were only present in my left eye. The bad news was that the blood vessels in my right eye were severely swollen and would probably rupture as well. I left the office that day with a patch over my left eye and a completely broken spirit.

I was completely crushed. I wondered exactly what was going to happen. I wondered if I was going to get my vision back in my left eye and if I was going to lose the vision I had left in my right eye. I felt like I only had half of my world. I was forced to wear that eye patch for two days. When those two days were up and I took the eye patch off, I expected to have my vision back. I expected to see normally again. I expected that big, black oil spill on the canvas of my life to be gone. It was not gone. That big, black oil spill on the canvas of my life was still there. I thought that was the worst of it. I thought that I would have this horrible black splotch in my vision forever and that I would just have to get used to it. I thought that it had gotten as bad as it was going to get. I thought that I would never have to go through that painful surgery again and could at least function close to normal since I still had the vision in my right eye. I thought wrong.

It was only about a week after I recovered from the surgery in my left eye that I began to see that little "fish" swimming around in my right eye. As soon as I saw it I knew what was happening. I panicked. I realized that this little "fish" swimming around in my visual field might just be the last thing I would ever see. I realized that I might be losing what vision that I had left. I could only see a tiny dot of the world out of my left eye. My right eye was really all that I had left. As I watched that "fish" get larger and larger my panic turned to dread. I knew my blood vessels had burst. I knew that I had to get to Dr. Gerber right away. I dropped what I was doing, got into my truck and rushed to Dr. Gerber's office while I could still see to get there. The "oil spill" on the canvas of my vision was taking over. I began to worry that I would not be able to see to get to the doctor's office. I began to pray fervently for the Lord to help me see to get help. I began to pray fervently for this darkness to stop growing. I began to pray fervently for this not to be real, but it was.

I had the same surgery on my right eye that very day. I gritted my teeth through the pain and prayed for a miracle this time. My miracle did not come. When my two days were up and the eye patch came off, my vision was not back. I was completely devastated. Over the next few weeks, I had four more surgeries to repair four more "bleeders" in my eyes. I became overwhelmed with a feeling of hopelessness. This hopelessness was coupled with fear. I had a fear of the surgery center. I had a fear of becoming blind for life. I had so many laser surgeries that I needed to have artificial vitreous fluid put into my eyes to try and tackle my blindness from a different perspective. That did not work either. Dr. Gerber finally gave up. My eye surgery was the last surgery that Dr. Gerber ever performed. Dr. Gerber declared me legally blind and referred me to the *Arizona Center for the Blind*.

I remember very well my conversations with a lady named Sheri who worked for the *Arizona Center for the Blind*. Sheri called me constantly and let me know that she had been through the same thing and now was completely blind but had learned to function quite well despite that fact. Was she serious? Was she really telling me that I was now a ***blind man***? I could not believe it! Dr. Gerber and this sympathetic voice on the phone named Sheri wanted me to accept the fact that my diabetes had caused me to go blind forever; they wanted me to be Gregg "the blind man with diabetes" Milliken. I refused. I refused to sign the papers that stated I was legally and completely blind. I refused to accept the fact that this disease had taken my sight away from me. I refused to return Sheri's phone calls. I refused to give up. I began to pray fervently. I began to pray fervently for a healing – a healing that I hoped would come very soon.

Blindness is almost indescribable. Once I lost sight in both of my eyes, I began to realize just how wonderful my world had been when I could see. I began to realize that I could no longer walk around my house without aid. Sometimes I would sit on the couch and as a result of habit pick up a magazine. Then I would realize that I could not read it. I had some sight left: a tiny pinhole that constantly drained my mental abilities as my brain constantly tried to enlarge it. Through that pinhole I saw many "what ifs." What if I never got my sight back? What if this is what God has in store for me for the rest of my life? What if I never see another sunset? What if I really need something? What if I am left all alone and I get lost because I cannot see where I am going? What if I never get to look in the mirror again? What if this darkness lasts forever?

At first, my blindness was just chaotic. Having diabetic retinopathy was a slam to my confidence, my strength, my psyche, and my spirituality. One of the most difficult things for me to do was just relax and make it through the day. That tiny pinhole that I had left was just enough to make me insane. I remember using that pinhole not just as a "what if", but as a ray of hope that I would one day regain all of my eyesight. I would sit for what seemed like hours and concentrate on that pinhole and wait for it to get larger. Sometimes I would look for so long that the pinhole would go away. At that point I would begin to panic and blink over and over until I realized that the pinhole of hope was indeed still there and that I had just stared in one spot for too long. It was driving me absolutely crazy to just have that small dot of what was once a full view of the world. I prayed constantly that the pinhole would somehow become larger and larger until one day I would really see again. I had to find my faith in order to maintain my sanity. I had to finally see that belief is much stronger than blindness. Although Dr. Gerber, my friends, and Sheri from the *Arizona Center for the Blind* had no faith in my regaining my eyesight, I was forced to have faith in order to survive. I was forced to reach deep inside of myself and find a way to make it through each and every day. I was forced to find the faith to face the day to day challenges of my new life with Jesus Christ by my side and with someone to guide me.

Being blind makes something as simple as walking around the house a ridiculous challenge. It is amazing what you take for granted when you can see it. Something as simple as eating was a challenge now that I was blind. Just imagine what it was like to try to use a knife! Tying my shoes was a challenge. Testing my blood glucose levels and taking my insulin injections was almost impossible. It had been difficult enough to give myself injections when I could see what I was doing, but now it was just guess work. I could not even see to measure out the proper amount of insulin. Dressing, eating, brushing my teeth, using the restroom (just try to close your eyes and aim!), getting a glass of water and just about any daily activity one does without thinking when they can see becomes a challenge when you go blind. Going out with my friends became a thing of the past. Up until the point that I lost my eyesight I was quite the socialite. I spent my days working and most of my evenings out with my friends until I lost my eyesight. Once I lost my eyesight, most my friends were not around anymore. I recall one day in particular when a friend I had not heard from in quite a few months called me and gave me the invitation to go out. I had to decline, and I proceeded to let him know that I was now legally blind. I will never forget the dead silence on the other end of the phone when I gave him the news that I was blind. The phone call ended shortly after that and I never heard from him again. Now I realized that not only did I have a disease, now I was "disabled." I began to feel more and more disabled as one by one my friends began to disappear. I began to feel alone in this darkness. I had only one or two friends that stuck by my side after I became blind. I am sure that it is difficult to remain friends with someone that cannot even see you. I will always be grateful to those that stuck by my side. They understood that if my eyesight never came back that I was still "Gregg" and that I still needed friends.

Being blind is very disconcerting. While I was blind I gained a new respect for blind people. They are the bravest people out there, trust me. While I was blind I constantly lived in fear. Since, of course, I was not born blind, I did not have the bravery that those who are born blind have. I was raised as a man that could see, so once I could not see I felt helpless. I could not go to the store. I could not cook a meal. I could not work out at the gym. I could not play tennis with my friends. I could not watch television or a movie. I could not read a magazine. I could not read my Bible. All I could do was sit and think and listen to the world around me. I began to spend my time meditating on God. I prayed fervently. I began to spend my time praying to God that I would regain my eyesight. I began meditating on what I could remember of the Bible. I began to realize that if I did not regain my eyesight that I would spend the rest of my life remembering what everything looks like and depending on someone else to tell me if anything changed. I could not even give myself my insulin injection at this point. I could not see my leg in order to inject the insulin into it. My life was very, very different and I felt very, very helpless.

One of the most difficult aspects of blindness for me was the boredom. It did not take me very long to begin to get ridiculously bored. I could no longer spend my time at the gym chiseling out my body into the physique that I had envisioned for years. I was in phenomenal shape at the time I went blind. I used to exercise for hours on end before I lost my eyesight. Now, I could not even see a dumbbell. I could no longer read the bodybuilding magazines that had given me the knowledge that I had needed to help control my diabetes. I could no longer drive to the gym five days a week and get the exercise that I so desperately needed in order to keep my body healthy. I could not even see my body and I completely lost the desire to be fit. I realized that I had taken for granted everything that God had given me up to this point in my life. I realized that everything I did from this point on was going to be a challenge, but that I better start being grateful for these challenges. I began to find my faith and trust the Lord more and more and pray to regain my eyesight.

The thing I missed the most was reading. Reading had been such an important part of my life for so long that I was not sure what to do without the ability. I had spent years reading bodybuilding magazines and supplement articles in order to learn how to make my body stronger and better able to cope with my diabetes. I missed reading my Bible. I missed reading and learning about my disease. I felt that if maybe I could see just enough to read I could learn how to beat this blindness. I often tried to pick up a magnifying glass and hold it close to that tiny pinhole that was my vision and attempt to read. But it was useless. I could not read. I could not even see. That tiny pinhole of light was just a cruel joke. I continued to have surgeries in the hopes of getting some of my vision back. So far, it was only hope.

Another thing I missed was vacation. Every year from the time I was a very young boy up until the time I went blind I went to San Diego, California on vacation with my family. For the past ten years or so I was a very physical person. I was a bodybuilder. I was in shape. I thoroughly enjoyed being in shape. I enjoyed riding bicycles. I enjoyed swimming in the ocean. I enjoyed hanging out on the beach and looking at the beautiful women. (I was young and single at the time.) I enjoyed just being physical and active and young. Vacation was one of the times when I felt normal. While I was on vacation I did not feel diseased. I felt attractive. I felt comfortable on the beach. Comfortable, that is, until I went blind. Now even more of my life had been taken away by my diabetes. I no longer felt comfortable on the beach. I could hear the ocean and I could smell the ocean, but I could not see it. I could feel the breeze hitting my face as it came off the ocean, but I could not see the waves. I could hear footsteps and giggles as women walked by, but I could not see them. I could not ride my bicycle down the boardwalk. I only knew that it was a sunny day on the beach because I could feel the sun beating down on my skin. I could not, however, see the sun or the clouds. This was no longer a vacation: it was misery. This darkness had ruined my vacations. This darkness felt like it had ruined everything. Instead of returning home from vacation feeling refreshed and revived, I returned home absolutely miserable.

Through this darkness I began to "see" people a little differently, so to speak. Being blind gave me a totally different outlook on life. When you cannot see what people look like, when you cannot see a facial expression, when you have no eyeballs staring back at your own you realize that the eyes do say so much and that the eyes truly are the "windows to the soul." When you cannot see anyone, you begin to realize just how much you judge another person based on looks. Now, all I had was the sound of a voice. I could no longer see if someone was happy, sad, angry, or content. I had to listen very closely to hear how a voice sounded so that I could "see" how someone was feeling in my mind. For the first time in my life "tone" of voice became important. I had to base everything on the tone of a person's voice. I had to decide a mood, a desire, a like, a dislike, happiness, sadness, impatience: all emotions based on tone of voice. (My wife will tell you that I still have issues with tone of voice.) It became amazing to me what you can hear in someone's voice when you cannot see their face. It absolutely blew me away to move from a "video" world to an "audio" world. Try it for just one day: turn off the television and live on only radio talk. Not music, radio *talk*. Try and hear just what people are trying to say without seeing them. If you really try this then you will realize what takes over in the life of the blind: imagination.

Without eyesight, imagination runs wild. Images form in your mind based on imagination and imagination is based on memory. I remembered what a sunset, a beautiful day, a full moon, and the ocean looked like and would just imagine them in my mind. At the end of the day I could just imagine the vision of the sunset over the mountains, I could even remember it, but I just could not see it. My dreams were much more vivid than they had ever been before while I was blind. It was as if my mind allowed me only to truly "see" in my dreams. I was full of memories of the things that I used to see and my mind played with those memories during my sleep. I remembered everything that I had done and I remembered what everything and everyone looked like. I would even dream about what I looked like, since I could no longer even see myself. I realized that I did have some advantage over those that had never had any eyesight: I had memories. I had the ability to use touch and memory to form images in my mind of how things should look. I remembered what everything looked like and I tried to use that as some conciliation to the fact that I may never see anything again.

While I was blind I began to wonder why this wretched disease called diabetes had to be my destiny. I began to wonder why God had taken my eyesight from me. For a long time I only lived in the past and I could not face the future. I was convinced that the greatest joys I had in life had been a direct result of my perfect eyesight. I did not understand how I was supposed to make it through the world by knocking my toes on street curbs and walking into walls. I did not understand why God had taken away my ability to read a magazine and study the Bible. I pitied myself for quite some time. Despite my self-pity, I tried to find joy somewhere. I enjoyed the smell of my mother's freshly baked cookies and the sound of the sprinklers coming on outside in the front yard. I sometimes would dig deep into my soul and try to find joy somewhere so that I could just listen to myself laugh. I would tell jokes to my mother so that I could listen to her laugh as well. My mother was wonderful while I was blind. I was forced to move back in with her since I could no longer take care of myself. She would tell me that my clothes did not match or that my hair looked terrible just to get a laugh out of me. Well, I hope she was trying to make me laugh. The point is she helped shed some joyous light into the miserable darkness of my world.

I want you to try and feel what I felt during this time. I urge you to cover up your eyes for twenty-four hours. Tape them up. Tie a bandana over them. Find some way to force yourself into darkness for just one day. Try to walk around without running into anything. Try to experience the fear that comes from not being able to see anything in your world. Are you afraid? Are you trying your hardest to remember where everything is so that you do not run into it? How do voices sound? Can you tell how someone is feeling just by the sound of their voice? Imagine not being able to take off the tape or the bandana or whatever you have chosen to use to cover your eyes. Imagine removing the eye patches after surgery – imagine just feeling the eye patches peeling off of your eyes – and then opening your eyes to darkness. Can you imagine? Can you really imagine? I began to feel a pity deep in my soul from the darkness of this devastating disease that I was plagued with at just nine years old. I had to find a way to see the world differently. I had to find a way to play the cards that God had dealt me. I had to find a way to see something positive in the wake of disaster.

I did learn to "see" the world a little differently while I was blind. I realized that things like a clean car and skin color are not important when you do not see them. I realized that I needed someone with me all the time so that I did not get hurt. I realized that I needed Jesus Christ in my life. I realized that without the Lord, nothing is worth it. I began to pray, and pray fervently. I found a renewed faith. I did not have to see anything in order to pray. I began to lean heavily on my faith as my world was enveloped in darkness. I realized that despite this darkness, my faith in the Lord would pull me through. I began to realize that my Lord was much bigger than my problems. I was definitely afraid, but I was not alone.

When my eye surgeries continued, it was with a renewed faith. I stirred up the confidence to go to the office of Dr. Sell and ask for another surgery. Dr. Sell had taken over for Dr. Gerber who had retired just after my last eye surgery. Dr. Sell was very confident, very positive, and I felt was very blessed by God. I felt that Dr. Sell was the surgeon and the chance that I had been praying for. Although I had already had more than twelve eye surgeries under Dr. Gerber and had been declared legally blind, Dr. Sell agreed to give my eyes one more try. Keep in mind that this was about fifteen years ago, and technology is not where it is today. At my initial consultation, Dr. Sell informed me that we had one shot at getting my vision back and he was going to take it. As I prepared for the surgery, I again prayed for God to give me back my vision and to guide the hand of this surgeon.

While I was blind, I had time to think of how my life was incomplete. I had never been married. I did not yet have children. I was not yet established in my career. I wanted to get back into bodybuilding. I wanted to be and have so many things that I wanted to SEE when I had them. My mother was taking care of me at the time, and she was wonderful. Again, my mother did everything that she could to keep me positive and keep my spirits up. She constantly reminded me that even if I never regained my eyesight that my life was not over, it was just different. My mother would hold my hand and take me for walks in our neighborhood. She knew how important exercise was to me, and she did her best to make sure that I got out of the house and could take walks or go to the gym. I had a friend that owned a gym that volunteered to help me around his gym when I wanted to go and exercise while I was blind. It was refreshing to have the ability to be normal at least for a few hours a week. Regardless, I continued to pray for a miracle. I continued to pray to God that this storm would blow over. Blindness as a result of diabetic retinopathy is like a storm: it flashes quickly like lightning, yet the rain continues. I prayed fervently that the rain of darkness would stop falling on me. I prayed that God was leading me to the right place at the right time. I continued to pray that Dr. Sell would be the man that would give me back my eyesight.

Throughout my twenties and well into my thirties, I was very naive. I did not realize that if I held my breath while I was lifting weights that I could pop the blood vessels in my eyes. (This was a bit of wisdom that Dr. Sell shared with me.) I also did not realize what a long shot it was for this final surgery to be successful. I kept praying and I had my faith and I was very patient. I do not know what the operating room looked like, but I am sure it was perfect. As soon as my mother walked me into the door of Dr. Sells' office, the nurses went to work. Dr. Sell had a staff that was absolutely amazing. They could tell that I was nervous, yet very hopeful. Once I was in the chair, I heard all the tools clanking and the nurses whisper and Dr. Sell let me know that he was about to begin the surgery. This time, there was no pain. What there was, however, was something that I can barely describe. What I "saw" while Dr. Sell was performing the surgery was absolutely amazing. All I remember seeing is rainbows of color dance across my visual field. I could not see any real "things" but I saw lines of colors that I had never seen before. I kept seeing

flashes of green and red and purple and yellow and blue. I was lying

there in this chair, probably laughing, at these amazing colors that

were dancing in front of my eyes. Due to my amazement, I was not

really listening to anything that the nurses and Dr. Sell were saying. I

was just lying there completely engrossed in what I was seeing. After

some time, the colors began to fade. Once the colors faded, I heard

Dr. Sell say very clearly to his staff, "Hurry and clean up my tools, I

have to get to the Sun's game."

I could not believe what I had just heard!! Either this was the

most shallow person ever to walk the face of the earth or the most

confident surgeon that was not even a little worried about what he had

just done. This man did not need a conference call, he did not need to

give me bad news, he was not freaking out and worrying about my

eyesight, he just needed to get to the Phoenix Sun's basketball game. I

was not sure how to take it. I was lying there listening to Dr. Sell

chuckle and rush his nurses so he could see a basketball game while

my future eyesight rested in his hands!! Was he really that shallow?

Or was he a great, great surgeon blessed by God?

After the surgery, I was wheeled back out to my mother to go home. I was told to go home and rest as much as I could and not to touch my eyes at all. As soon as my medication wore off, the pain began. I was in unbelievable pain! My eyes were aching worse than anything had ever ached in my entire life. On top of that, my eyes were itching so bad that I wanted to scream. I remember the nurses telling me that there were stitches in my eyes and that they would be somewhat uncomfortable; but I was not ready for how badly my eyes itched!! It was insane! The hardest thing that I ever had to do was NOT touch my eyes. Luckily, I only had to deal with that for one night, and I was due to go back the next morning. I believe it was Saturday morning. (I am guessing that it was Saturday, since the Suns normally play on Friday night.) I was unbelievably nervous and completely exhausted from dealing with the pain and itching in my eyes all night. I was also excited. I was excited about opening my eyes. I was hoping that all of my prayers had been answered. I was hoping that I was finally getting my miracle.

When the bandages came off, I got my miracle. **I COULD SEE!!!** Images were forming in front of my eyes every time I blinked them! I could not believe it! I had one chance – once chance at regaining my eyesight and I took it and it worked!! The more that I blinked the more I could see. The only color I could see at first was red – blood red. I did not even care that the only color I could see was red. I was so happy that I could see that I would have been happy seeing in red forever. After I blinked a few more times, I suddenly realized what I could see through the red: I could see that everything was UPSIDE DOWN. What had happened? I was beginning to panic again. I was suddenly thinking that my world was literally turned upside down forever! I began speaking very quickly and nervously to Dr. Sell in order to let him know what I saw. Dr. Sell quickly eased my fears. He let me know that what I was seeing was perfectly normal. He let me know that God had given me a wonderful brain that will adjust to the surgery and turn everything right side up again. I thought that sounded a little bit crazy, but I believed him. I could see more than I had seen in such a long time that I knew that this was my miracle.

I COULD SEE AGAIN! Even though my world was red and upside down, I COULD SEE!! I was no longer a blind man. I remember sitting in that chair listening to Dr. Sell when he told me that the surgery was a complete success and that I will never have any more "bleeders" in my eyes. He did not have to tell me – I already knew. He told me that by the end of the day my world turn right side up again, and in a few days the color would correct itself and I would see normally. He told me that I will never go blind again. Dr. Sell told me that I could rip up the paperwork for the *Arizona Center for the Blind*. I could not believe my ears, or my eyes. **I could see**. I could see clearly. I could see everything. My eyesight was back! I felt like a new man. I felt like I had finally beaten a part of my disease for good. I knew that this was my miracle. This was my moment. This was my victory. I had defeated diabetic retinopathy. I was a champion. This battle with blindness was finally over; and I had won. Was it the skill of the doctor? Was it my faith? Was it my will to conquer this disease? I do not know what it was – but it was a miracle. My miracle.

To this day I appreciate all of the things that I can see. To this day I remember the innate joy I felt when I awoke that first morning with my complete eyesight and looked out the window and could see God's beautiful world. I will never take my eyesight for granted again. I will never take for granted the breathtaking smile that I see on my wife's face every morning when she wakes me up. I will never take for granted the sweet, beautiful faces of my children. I will never let another day go by without reading *The Bible*. I will always appreciate being able to see a movie. I will never again take for granted the beauty of the Grand Canyon or a simple sunset. I will never underestimate what this disease can do to my body again. I will never forget the amazing feeling of coming out of the darkness into the beauty of sight. I am a man that had lost both of his eyes and was granted the amazing gift of getting them back. The canvas of my life is fresh and new again. I will never underestimate the power of God. I am a champion. I am a survivor. I have overcome blindness. And I am a diabetic.

Overcoming blindness gave me new hopes and new dreams for my life. I knew that I could now harness my strength and with God by my side that I could accomplish my dreams. God had given me a new beginning and I was ready to take this newness of life and work toward the future that I had always dreamed of.

Chapter Six

A New Beginning

Once I regained my eyesight, I began to have many new dreams for my life. I felt invincible. I now knew that, through faith, I could conquer anything. One dream that I wanted to bring to reality was the dream of becoming a police officer. Just like most boys, as a child I had wanted to be a police officer when I grew up.

At the time, I was a groundskeeper for the City of Phoenix. I had fantastic health insurance, which was of the utmost importance with diabetes. The City supported me while I was blind and I was able to return to work as usual once I regained my eyesight. My coworkers had donated their vacation time to me as well so that I would be able to return to work when I was healed. Everyone who knew me knew that I was not going to accept being handicapped; and they knew that I would be back. They were right. I was welcomed back with open arms. I am still grateful to everyone that donated their time and had faith in me. I was truly blessed, and I am still blessed today.

While I was a groundskeeper, I worked hard, but I wanted to be more. In the past, I had been told that I could not be a police officer because I had type 1 diabetes. Since that time, the American Diabetes Association and the Americans with Disabilities Act had come on strong to employers so that those of us with diabetes could no longer be discriminated against. Now that I knew that I had a chance, I began to train. And I do not mean train like I had in the past; I mean I trained with a new purpose. I hiked, I lifted weights, and I ran for miles six days a week. I also took classes on the weekends that would help me in my quest to become a police officer. I was ready. I looked healthy. I was strong. To everyone around me, I was normal again. It was as if the blindness had never occurred and everyone forgot that I had diabetes. I took the utmost care of myself and it began to show like it never had before. I took on the responsibility to work as hard as I could to get the job that I had wanted since I was a small child. I was working toward my dream. I had already defeated the effects of diabetes once and I was not going to let diabetes stop me from fulfilling my dream.

When I applied to the police academy, I was required to pass a field test. This field test basically included physical fitness skills and endurance. I passed with flying colors. The run was about a mile and a half, and my blood glucose level amazingly remained stable the whole time. I had finally figured out that I needed to fill by body with carbohydrates before a workout and I did just that. Due to my excellent scores on the field test, I was granted an interview. I just could not believe it! I was confident, I was excited, and I was finally where I worked so hard to be. The department was very pleased with my interview, and I was instantly accepted into the police academy. Wow! I could not believe it! This was a dream of mine coming true before my eyes. As I was shaking hands with the interviewer I was absolutely beaming. I was finally there. Then there was the scary news: I had to take a physical. I knew that during the physical it would be discovered that I had diabetes. I was a little afraid, but I knew that my field test scores would prove that I could do the job despite my disease. Then I was delivered the news that made my heart skip a beat: in order to pass the physical I had to pass a vision test. This is when the success of all of those eye surgeries and all of those prayers would be put to the test.

When the day of the physical came, I was a little nervous. I was given tons of paperwork to fill out, and I did so honestly. I was in amazing shape. No one could look at me and tell that I had any type of disease. My body was nothing but muscle and I kept my diabetes under excellent control. I did divulge the fact that I have diabetes, but not a word was said to me about it. Once I filled out the paperwork, the first thing I was required to do was take the vision test. I was required to take the vision test WITHOUT MY GLASSES. Before I took that test I closed my eyes and prayed. I prayed to God for those surgeries to have been complete, for my eyesight to be truly restored just as I felt it had been. I prayed for God to continue my miracle and for this disease to not disappoint me again. I opened my eyes and took the vision test. I did everything I was told. First my left eye was tested, then my right eye, and then both eyes. When it was over I looked to the face of the nurse for a clue as to my results. She looked at me, smiled, and let me know that I passed with flying colors. My prayers had just been answered! After blindness, after countless eye surgeries, after months of fear and darkness and fervent prayer I passed that vision test with FLYING COLORS. My excitement was above comprehension. I still had my miracle. Once again, I beat my disease and my life was beginning anew.

Once I was in the academy, I began to have some problems with my blood glucose levels. The long runs were the worst. I tried to make sure that I had plenty of carbohydrates in my body to make it through the long runs without needing sugar, and most of the time this method worked for me. Sometimes, however, I would eat too many carbohydrates and end up with my legs feeling like lead and dying of thirst. Despite the effects of my disease I persevered. I made it. Since we had to endure so much physical activity, I had to make sure that I had plenty of sugar and carbohydrates on hand. I still did not mention that I had diabetes to my Recruit Training Officer (RTO). My RTO and most of my classmates just assumed that I ate so much because I was a bodybuilder. They would see the massive size of my chest, arms, and legs and assume that it took quite a few calories to feed those muscles. I let them think it. I did not want anyone to know that I had a weakness. I was at the top. I was in the police academy. I was strong. I was on my way to becoming the best of the best. We were the ones that took care of the weak – not the ones with weaknesses. I relied on my knowledge of my disease and my faith in God to get me through. It worked. I kept my stress level low and my blood glucose level as normal as I could. I was a complete success. I was proud. I was, again, living my dream despite my disease.

Just before I entered the police academy, I got married. And along with the natural order of things, I became the proud father of two beautiful baby girls. You cannot imagine my innate joy at being able to see the faces of my daughters. Sometimes I still just look at them, thankful to God for the ability to see their beautiful faces. As they became a little older, I began to realize the danger of the career that I had chosen. For this, and a few other reasons, including divorce and child care issues, I left my dream job and returned to my position as groundskeeper for the City of Phoenix. This was one of the most difficult decisions I ever made. I had defeated blindness and diabetes and all the odds to land a job as a police officer, but my daughters were much more important to me than my job. The decision I made to stay with the city, however, made it possible for me to keep my health insurance and left the door open to many other opportunities.

While working as a groundskeeper, I began to take notice of the Park Rangers that I constantly saw around the city. I befriended one of them, and as we got to know each other, I began to mention that I had been in the police department. He could not believe that I had gone from police officer to groundskeeper. He knew quite a few police officers and knew what the academy had entailed. He noticed that I was in phenomenal shape and he suggested that I interview for the position of Park Ranger. I would still be working for the city, and I would have the ability to stay physically active while on the job. He assured me that it was much safer than a career in the police department, and that the benefits package, including health insurance and retirement, was definitely better than that of a groundskeeper. So, I took his advice and began researching a career as a Park Ranger.

When I first attempted to interview, I was rejected. I was a little shocked that I would be refused since I was formerly with the police department. I was told that thousands apply for that job every month and that I had a very small chance of being chosen. I was told, at the City of Phoenix Career Center, to try and get a job with the American Diabetes Association since I had diabetes. I was told that would have a much better chance getting a job with them than I would of having a chance at becoming a Park Ranger. I was disappointed, to say the least, but I did not give up. I let them know that I would keep applying for the job until I got it. I persevered, worked hard, and refused to give up. Time to time I would reapply for the Park Ranger position, and every time I was refused an interview. I did not give up. I continued to work hard as a groundskeeper for the city and hope that they noticed. I was very healthy at the time. Working as a groundskeeper kept me in shape and allowed me to meet quite a few people. Although I had gone from groundskeeper to police officer back to groundskeeper, I was very successful, well-liked by my superiors, and had been faithful to the city. This must have helped my cause. After applying every few months for an entire year, I was finally granted the chance to interview for the position of Park Ranger. I could not believe it when I got the call. Was I really going to be lucky enough to live out a second dream? Was I going to be able to, again, pass a physical challenge with diabetes and land a dream career? Circumstances almost prevented it.

Just about a week before my interview, I became ill. It began as just a cold but quickly advanced into something worse. Now, if you know anything about diabetes, then you know that any type of illness can be serious. A common cold can, before you know it, turn into pneumonia and land you in the hospital. When the body of someone with type 1 diabetes is attempting to fight infection, blood glucose levels rise dramatically. When the day of my interview came, I was sicker than ever. Instead of getting better, my cold was getting worse and worse. My blood glucose levels where so high that I could barely even function. I was forced to take large amounts of insulin just to keep my blood glucose low enough to function. I did not have the energy to exercise, and I felt like I did not have the strength to get off of the couch. When the morning of my interview came, I prayed. I prayed for God again to give me the strength that I needed to succeed again. I prayed for a healing. I prayed for mercy. I prayed for yet another victory in my daily battle with diabetes.

I found the strength to get up off the couch to go to my interview. It was raining. It was cold. And I was extremely ill. I was fevered. I was tired. I was just sick. However, I chose to pile on the insulin and try to do my best. Part of the interview required hiking up a mountain trail and naming the desert plants that were along the trail. I could not believe that I had to do this in the rain while I was sick. I prayed once again, took a large dose of insulin, and began to hike.

About halfway up the trail I began to feel fantastic. I do not know if it was the insulin, the fact that I had got up off the couch and was moving around, or if it was the grace of God; but I felt amazing. I found a new energy. I sped up. I hiked to the top of that mountain trail, down again, and passed the physical and written portions of my interview with flying colors. Again, I had found my miracle. God had allowed me to beat this disease one more time and become a success.

When the physical portion of the interview was over, I was put into a van with some supervisory personnel to ride back to the Ranger Station. To my surprise, one of the supervisors was an old friend of mine! God could not have put me in a better place at a better time. The interview concluded in the van, and I was more confident than ever. I knew that God had blessed me once again. I knew that I was again going to have the chance to be at the top of my game. I was going to be a Park Ranger. I just knew it.

Sure enough a few days later, I got the call. I was beaming. I was accepted into the Park Ranger program for the City of Phoenix. This was another dream come true. On my way home from work that evening, I thanked God. My scarred up eyes cried tears of joy that day. I was overjoyed that I had beaten the odds once again. I was at the top. I was about to enter the Ranger academy. I was going to be a Park Ranger. My life was turning from a life of disappointment due to my disease to a life of fulfillment despite my disease. I was now a man who had overcome. I overcame hypoglycemia that left me hospitalized as a child. I overcame comas due to hyperglycemia. I overcame sickness. I overcame blindness. I overcame diabetes. I had diabetes; but it no longer had me. I received my fifteen year service award from the City of Phoenix Parks and Natural Resources Division in 2008: proof that I am still overcoming.

I cannot express how important it is to take care of your health in order to overcome this disease. I would not be where I am today and I would not be on top of my disease if I did not take care of my body. Not only does exercise keep me strong, but I know in order to control diabetes, I have to control my diet.

Chapter Seven

Diet

I cannot leave out the important issue of diet. As a diabetic, whether type 1 or type 2, it is imperative that one follow a strict diet. As a child, my mother chose my diet for me. The only major thing that I recall is that I did not like peas and I did not like the fact that she would severely limit my sugar intake. Like most children would do, I assume, I fed my peas to the dog and ate sweets in secret. My mother did the best that she could to make sure that I got the best nutrition possible; especially considering that she was a nurse and was very well educated in the particulars of diabetes. I thank my mother now for limiting the amount of sweets I was allowed, although at the time it truly did seem like torture.

Looking back, I craved sweets almost twenty-four hours a day. I had myself convinced that I loved sweets and that I just could not live without them. Once I finally grew up and changed my thought patterns, I began to crave life much more than I craved sweets. I began to realize that if I wanted to live a long and healthy life then I needed to follow a strict diet like my mother had forced upon me. (Mom knows best, right?) It was so much easier to stay on my diet when I was not stressed, I exercised, and I was focused on becoming healthy.

One way to have and maintain a healthy diet is to realize that every day is a new day. I love a new day. If I cheated a little the day before, it was always easy to begin anew. After the eight hour cleanse that your body gets when you sleep (anyone with diabetes should sleep AT LEAST eight hours a night) it is wonderful to wake up and put healthy food in your body. Good nutrition early in the day makes for the insulin need to be much less during the rest of the day. I have found it very beneficial to drink fresh juice at the beginning of the day. I have a home juicer, and I drink homemade juice every morning. I would recommend juicing to everyone, especially diabetics. It is a wonderful way to begin the day with proper nutrition and blood glucose management. Once the desire is in the heart to be healthy and beat this disease, good eating habits will follow.

Another important part of a healthy diet is fiber. Fiber keeps your body cleansed and helps with absorption. Absorption becomes very important to a diabetic when they are ingesting glucose during a hypoglycemic reaction. If fiber is supplemented on a daily basis, it is much easier for the body to absorb the foods that are ingested. This, again, is something that a person with diabetes should take very seriously.

Green tea is another important dietary staple for diabetes. Green tea is an antioxidant that aides in weight loss. It is not a secret that diabetes is now becoming an epidemic in this country due to the obesity rate. So many Americans could cure their type 2 diabetes if they would just control their weight. Although type 1 diabetes does not have a cure, I am a testimony to the fact that successful blood glucose management can only be achieved when the body is kept at a healthy weight. In order to maintain a healthy weight, it is important for anyone, diabetics included, to stop eating so much packaged food and start eating fruits and vegetables. It is easy to keep yourself prepared. I take a small cooler wherever I go, and I keep it stocked with vegetables, fruits, and, of course, insulin and fast acting glucose. That little cooler can save my life and keep me from going to the fast food restaurant for a snack when I am hungry. It may be what quite a few people consider a little inconvenient, but I would much rather be a little inconvenienced than overweight and out of control with my blood glucose levels. Wouldn't you?

Having diabetes takes discipline. Anyone with diabetes will tell you that. You have to have the discipline to say no to sweets. You have to have the discipline to learn how to count carbohydrates and sugars. You have to have the discipline to test your blood glucose levels up to eight times a day to make sure that you are in the "normal" range. Every decision made throughout the day revolves around this disease. The discipline that is required to just keep this disease from killing you is more than enough discipline to maintain a nutritious diet. Anyone with diabetes has the strength within them to have the control it takes to make the most of this disease and follow a proper diet.

In order to maintain this diet, I hope that diabetics remember to always put their disease first and to let everyone in their lives know that this disease comes first. It is impossible to have control without support. Everyone in your life needs to know that you WILL follow a nutritious diet and that you WILL need glucose (or sweets) when you have a hypoglycemic reaction. Everyone in my life knows that I need to have three things on my person all the time: my blood-glucose monitor, insulin, and fast-acting glucose. End of story. In today's world there is no reason why every diabetic would not have those three essentials within their grasp ALL THE TIME. Water is another essential, but nothing like insulin and fast-acting glucose. The best way to always have these things is to educate everyone around you about your disease. There is no reason to be shy or embarrassed. If someone does not understand, explain it to them. Let everyone know what you need. You deserve that. You require that. You have the strength to find a way.

When I went blind, I really began to question my diet. I could not help but wonder if it was my fault. I began to wonder if the blindness was my fault because I would sneak around and eat sugars that I did not need. It was so easy at that time to look down upon myself for all of the mistakes that I had made in the past. At that time I did not appreciate the fiber in an apple or the omega-3 in a piece of salmon. I did not realize that one box of prepackaged food had enough sodium to meet the maximum daily requirement of such for one whole week. I did not change overnight, but my blindness made me realize that I could do so much better. I realized that I had to change. I had to take steps – they were baby steps – but they were steps. Once I regained my eyesight, that day was the first day of the rest of my life.

God had given me my eyesight back and I began to eat the foods that He provided for us on this earth: fruits, vegetables, red meats, and eggs. I also began to take supplements like l-argenine and l-glutamine. Although I am not a doctor and I am not a scientist, I am a Certified Personal Trainer and I know how much good these amino acids will do the body – especially the body of a diabetic. Not to mention I have had diabetes for almost forty years. Challenge me. Look it up. But do not doubt that this can be the first day of the rest of your life and you can use proper diet and supplementation to aid in the control of your disease. Proper diet and supplementation can change the life of a diabetic. Energy can be gained and weight can be lost and blood glucose levels can be controlled. I have recovered from blindness and I will never eat badly again due to that little "fish" that swam in front of my eye that day. Was my blindness due to poor diet and poor blood glucose control? It is possible. Do I want to risk becoming blind again? Not a chance. Therefore, I follow a healthy diet…just in case. If you have diabetes, I urge you to follow a healthy diet as well. I do not want you to go blind: it is scary, it is empty, and it is preventable. Good nutrition can prevent that little "fish" from swimming into your life. Think about it.

Not only is it important to follow a healthy diet, it is of the utmost importance to educate yourself on the technology associated with your disease. I have seen insulin therapy and diabetes evolve in leaps and bounds in my lifetime. My doctors and my constant strive to maintain my health and control of this disease have caused me to learn so much about diabetes and stay on the very edge of technology. We are on the verge of a cure, and the technology that is available to manage diabetes is constantly improving.

Chapter Eight

Insulin Therapy and Technology

Diabetes management has come a long way since I was nine years old. I firmly believe the days of the orange and the syringe are over. As a child, I took only one insulin injection in the morning and hoped that it worked effectively all day. The insulin used at that time was animal insulin, and it did not work as well to regulate blood glucose levels as the insulin does today. The first synthetic insulin created using human DNA was not introduced until 1982. By that time, I had already suffered from diabetes for ten years and I noticed a remarkable difference in my body once I switched to human insulin. The new insulin worked much better with my body and I was so excited to experience a positive change.

The sticks that I was forced to use as a child to monitor whether my blood glucose was high or low were extremely inconvenient. I recall that when I was feeling the effects of hyperglycemia, I was told to use these "sticks" to see my blood glucose level was in fact reaching a dangerously high level. These "sticks" were small, plastic sticks about the size of my pointer finger. They had a strip on one side that, when it came in contact with urine, measured the amount of ketone in my body. Ketone is an acid that the body of a diabetic produces when the body is burning too much fat and the diabetes has become out of control. Too much ketone in the body of a diabetic can lead to a coma, which happened to me on more than one occasion. Part of this is probably due to the fact that I found the ketone testing sticks inconvenient to use – I had to find a place to urinate, wait three to five minutes after urinating on the stick to check the results, and I had to keep the bottle of these sticks with me all the time because it contained the color chart that I needed to know at what level the ketone in my body had reached. It was very difficult for me to match the stick color to the chart color as well. Not to mention, I was a child, I was newly diagnosed, and I was completely embarrassed to use these sticks at school. It was beyond my strength level as a child to use these sticks in front of my friends, especially considering that most of them did not even know that I had a disease. This was just one of so many new tasks that I was given as a young child that I truly was not ready to tackle. I am so grateful that technology has come up with something better.

Before I was lucky enough to have a blood glucose monitor and human insulin, I was forced to basically be my own doctor. I would have to guess by my body signals if I was normal, hypoglycemic, or hyperglycemic and treat myself accordingly. Again, the insulin that I had as a child was animal insulin, and it was not very effective. Sometimes the injection that I took in the morning lasted all day long for me, and sometimes it did not. Now, diabetics are lucky enough to have Humulin (human insulin), fast-acting, and slow acting insulin. It is amazing to me how far the treatment of this disease has come in these thirty seven years. Fast acting insulin and slow acting insulin are both now available. Not only are they available, they are available in the form of a "penlet" that takes the stress out of using a vial and a syringe. When using a syringe and a vial of insulin, it is imperative to make sure that the insulin is drawn out of the vial with no bubbles, and then injected into the body before bubbles form in the syringe. Do you really think that a child could do that? Of course not. Problems such as that are the reasons why it has been so difficult for children to take control of their diabetes. With the insulin "penlet,' the insulin is ready to be injected. A small needle is screwed onto the tip of the "penlet" and then discarded after use. There is even a device on the end that allows the user to click the pen to the number of units of insulin to be injected. It is amazing, simple, and can be used easily by a child. Insulin therapy is better controlled with the technology of better insulin delivery.

It took me many years to learn how my metabolism worked. I did not understand through most of my childhood exactly what it meant that my blood glucose level was too high or too low. Without a blood glucose monitor, I had never seen a number that correlated with my blood glucose level. All I knew was that the little plastic stick could be too red sometimes (I was supposed to be in the "pink" all the time) and if it was I knew that I needed some insulin. The amount of insulin I needed to take, of course, was merely guesswork. Although the first home glucose monitor was invented in 1971 (the year prior to my diagnosis), it did not become available to the public until the late 1980's.

By the time I received my first blood glucose monitor, I was well on my way to understanding my metabolism and insulin needs. When my doctor first mentioned the blood glucose monitor, I was not sure what he was speaking of. My doctor told me that there was now a "blood tester" available and that he was going to give me one. What?

A blood tester? I had never even heard of such a thing. I thought that it sounded a little crazy, but I agreed to give it a try. I am so thankful that I did. The blood glucose monitor changed my life completely. I have to admit that I was quite skeptical at first. I did not want to prick my finger – it was bad enough that I had to take injections. Not to mention that if I carried this monitor around I would no longer be able to hide the fact that I had a disease from others. Of course, the monitor was much larger then than it is today (and required a much larger drop of blood), but it was amazing to begin to see a number correlate with the way that I felt. With a blood glucose monitor, I could finally understand where my blood glucose level was supposed to be, at what level it was when I felt hypoglycemic, at what level it was when I felt hyperglycemic, and how much insulin I needed to take in order to enjoy a meal. I cannot express how much better my life became when I was able to test my blood glucose level. At first, I became somewhat obsessed with this new knowledge of my blood glucose level and tested nonstop. I checked my blood glucose level at least every hour when I first obtained my monitor. I do not check it quite as often now, of course, but I know how amazing that it truly is to be able to know my blood glucose level at any given moment.

Today, the monitors are so small that they fit in the hand of a child and the drop of blood required to sample is miniscule. Diabetes management is within complete reach thanks to this innovative technology.

Another amazing invention in diabetes management has been the insulin pump. The first insulin pump was introduced in 1979, but was so large that it had to be carried in a backpack. Thankfully, they are no longer that inconvenient. My first insulin pump, which I first used about ten years ago, was very small, yet still very inconvenient. The actual pump that was programmable and delivered whatever amount of insulin that I programmed it to deliver, was attached to my body by a tube. This tube was inserted into my skin with a needle similar to the needles used to inject IV's. In order to use this pump, I had to program the pump to "prime" (put insulin into the tube), inject the needle and tubing into my skin, and then test to be sure that the tubing was inserted correctly. No only was this painful, the tubing would often be torn loose from the injection site, which would force me to have to set it up all over again. As a Park Ranger, I had an extremely difficult time using this insulin pump because the duty belt that I wear on the job would get caught on the tubing and pull it out.

After less than a year struggling with this pump, I went back to injecting insulin. However, another innovation with the insulin pump has given me another blessing with my disease and a new freedom. I now have the luxury of a wireless, tubeless insulin pump. Yes, I said wireless. And, yes, I said tubeless. Instead of giving myself injections, I now use the OmniPod Insulin Management System. This system delivers insulin through an extremely small, waterproof, wireless pump that is controlled by a small, Personal Diabetes Manager (PDM) device. This PDM device not only controls the amount of insulin that goes into my body, but it also helps me count carbohydrates your meals and tests blood glucose levels. It is amazing! The "pod" just sticks to my body, and once I program the PDM, the tube is automatically injected into my body so that I do not have to use any needles on my own. Can you believe it? Technology has come so far. I program my PDM to deliver insulin 24 hours a day, and then to deliver insulin based on the carbohydrate content of each of my meals. I have the best control of my diabetes with this device than I have had in my entire life with this disease. I do not have any tubes or wires to get tangled up in, and the PDM calculates my insulin needs and had a built in blood glucose tester. I would certainly suggest the OmniPod Insulin Management System to anyone with diabetes, but especially to children that have been diagnosed with type 1 diabetes. This system is ridiculously simple to use, and could mean so much to a child that is afraid of injections and embarrassed to test their blood glucose levels. If you have diabetes, be sure and ask your doctor about the OmniPod, or go to www.MyOmniPod.com for more information.

It is unbelievable how far the technology behind diabetes management has come. I have gone from beef insulin to human insulin, from Ketosticks to blood glucose monitors, and from one large injection a day to many injections a day. Now I take no injections at all because I have gone from a bulky insulin pump with a long tube to a completely tube and wire free insulin management system that even counts my carbohydrates! God has blessed so many lives with the wisdom of invention.

I cannot express enough how important it is to be educated about this disease if you suffer from it. I have made it a point to educate myself about my disease due to the fact that I learned at a very young age that doctors do not always share all of the information that they have, nor are they always up to date with innovative technologies.

Unfortunately, we live in a society where drug companies and health insurance companies control health care. The company with the most clout basically controls health care directives. Not to mention, if your doctor is not up to date on the most innovative and recent technological advances in diabetes care, you may be inadvertently missing out on better diabetes management. I have to say that most of the people that I speak to with my disease are not even aware that the insulin pump that I use exists. I heard about the OmniPod on a diabetes website, but when I spoke to my doctor about it, he had never heard of it. He mentioned that there were plenty of other insulin pumps out there that worked wonderfully, but he had not heard of this new wireless, tubeless pump. He also added that such an insulin pump would probably cost my insurance company a large amount of money. Fortunately, I have become a strong advocate for treating my disease and I have also become strong enough to demand the best treatment that exists for diabetes. I am so thankful that I am. I am now living with the best Insulin Management System on the market, and my doctor is now suggesting it to all of his patents that are approved for pump therapy. Again, I cannot express to you how important it is to be educated. Read books. Join websites that support diabetes research. Familiarize yourself with legislation involving the research and development of the management and treatment of this devastating disease. That is the difference between controlling diabetes and letting it control you.

Chapter Nine

Inspiration

Inspiration for anyone with diabetes happens in one or two ways. First, it is extremely rewarding to perform just as well, if not better, than someone who does not have the disease. It is even more rewarding when that person is complaining about how hard life is, how difficult the task the both of you are performing is, etc. Even as a child I had so many things happen to me that were inspiring, but they became even more inspiring due to the fact that I am living with diabetes. I always went out of my way to help others instead of being the one that needed help.

It is important to remember that someone with diabetes that takes the time to learn about their disease and take proper care of themselves is taking the time to save a life. Every single day your life rests in your hands when you suffer from diabetes. It takes a discipline, strength, and faith in God to conquer this disease on a daily basis. It is a daily struggle, but it is a struggle that can be overcome. The struggle with diabetes can be a struggle of success, and must be more about success that about failure. Those of us with diabetes may have started out weak, but this disease makes us strong. It takes strength to give yourself injections everyday, no matter how old that you are. It takes strength to prick your finger and to count carbohydrates and to let someone know when you desperately need glucose, even if they do not understand.

Believe it or not, diabetes has helped me develop my character. Without this disease, I probably would have gone through life on autopilot just like everyone else. Without this disease, I probably would not take such good care of my body, exercise regularly, and follow a proper diet. Not to mention the knowledge that I have gained about my body, how it works, what nutrients I need, and so much more that I would have never even attempted to learn if I did not have this disease. How many people without diabetes really understand what their pancreas does? How about beta cells? Diabetes not only shaped my character, it allowed to learn so much more than I would have learned if I did not have this disease.

I am so thankful to God that I am still going as strong as I am after having this disease for nearly forty years. I used to whine about my disease, but that is a thing of the past. I am so thankful to God every time that my blood tests such as my A1C have normal results. I am so thankful to God every time that I help someone move heavy furniture or help a lost hiker find their way back to the trail. I am so thankful to God every time I open my eyes and can actually see. Proper nutrition and intelligent living have given me an edge on this disease that not everyone has. If you suffer from diabetes, I encourage you to learn as much as you can about it. Although this disease cannot be cured, it can definitely be overcome through knowledge and understanding. No one has to be in a coma, no one has to guess at their glucose levels anymore, and no one has to go blind. Educate yourself. It is the only way to conquer this disease.

So many people do not realize how often diabetics truly feel close to death or how close to eternity we truly are every time that we go to sleep. I have to take a moment and just thank God for my wife. She is there beside me every time I wake with hypoglycemia and need help. She has kept me alive on many occasions by just waking up and force-feeding me glucose. I know that God has put her in my life for a reason and I again thank Him for that.

I can remember over the course of the last thirty-seven years having many hypoglycemic reactions and not having any form of glucose with me. Those were the scary times. I would sweat, my heart would pound, I would get confused, I would get nauseous, and it would become harder by the second to survive this thing called "diabetes". That is still one of the most difficult aspects of this disease for me: preventing hypoglycemia. However, that is just one of the many aspects of this disease that plague me twenty-four hours a day, seven days a week.

As a Park Ranger, it is even more important for me to make sure that I have enough glucose to get through the day. With a ten to twelve hour shift, constant hiking, and numerous mountain rescues it is important for me to have plenty of glucose on hand. I am still so proud and amazed that I was even able to obtain my position as Park Ranger with this disease. I would like to share a story of a particular mountain rescue that just proved to me that, again, God put me in this position for a purpose.

My partner and I were patrolling Camelback Mountain in Phoenix, Arizona. If you live in Arizona then you know that Camelback Mountain is one of the most popular hiking areas in the state. There are numerous trails that challenge hikers of all fitness levels. This being a preserve, there is no artificial lighting along the trails; therefore, Park Rangers constantly patrol this mountain in the daylight and especially in the dark.

One particular day, a man named Earl Baker had decided to hike to the top of Camelback Mountain for his eightieth birthday. He recalls beginning the hike around noon, which is in the hottest part of the day here in the Arizona desert.

Just prior to dusk, my partner and I decided to hike up Camelback Mountain as part of our patrol and make sure that all of the hikers were on their way down the trails. It is common knowledge that it is easy to get lost after dark, so most hikers time it so that they are off of the mountain prior to sunset. As we prepared to hike up the mountain, I grabbed my flashlight just in case we were still on the mountain after dark ourselves. Due to my diabetes, I always wear a "fanny pack" on my hip when I go hiking on the job. In my "fanny pack" I carry insulin, snacks, water, and fast-acting glucose. I carry snacks that are high in sugar and carbohydrates so that if I begin to feel hypoglycemic during my hike I can simply ingest some form of glucose. I have learned over the years (of course, the hard way) that if I am to be doing any type of physical activity that I need to be prepared for my blood glucose level to drop during or immediately after the activity. Not to mention that it would be pretty embarrassing for a Park Ranger to have to be rescued from the top of a mountain because he was unprepared. So, I was loaded with my flashlight, cell phone, and fanny pack as my partner and I began to hike up the trail.

On the way to the top of the mountain, we passed Earl Baker. At the time I did not know his name or his age, but I did know that he looked somewhat exhausted. My partner and I stopped and asked him if he was okay or if he needed any help down the mountain. Mr. Baker insisted that he was perfectly fine and that he would finish his hike down the mountain unaided. My partner and I took note of his condition, and continued to hike to the top of Camelback Mountain directing hikers down trail since sunset was approaching. On the way down the mountain, my partner and I were speaking to hikers, clearing the trail, and letting everyone know that they needed to be off the trail by nightfall. As it began to get dark, I began to wonder about the older gentleman that we had passed on the way up the mountain. Although he had said that he was alright, I just could not get him off of my mind.

This particular trail at Camelback Mountain is a difficult hike. There are quite a few slide areas, boulders to climb, rocky areas, steep climbs, rattlesnakes, and just about any other hazard you could imagine on a mountain preserve in the desert. As my partner and I made it about halfway down the mountain, we noticed a tiny LED light shining from the face of a large boulder. As we got a little closer to it, we realized that the light was coming from the hat of the gentleman that we had passed on the way up. He was standing flat against the face of the boulder. He was breathing heavily and looked as if he might be seconds from unconsciousness. We began speaking to this man, and he introduced himself as Earl Baker. We attempted to call for help on the radio, but soon realized that the battery on the radio had died. (Okay, I did forget to charge it the night before.) Cell phones do not carry a signal on Camelback Mountain, so my partner and I had no choice but to get Mr. Baker down the mountain on our own. Luckily, I had my "fanny pack" fully loaded, so I gave Mr. Baker some water and a snack high in carbohydrates so that he could regain enough of his strength to be able to be guided down the mountain. While he was eating, my partner and I had the most interesting conversation with Mr. Baker. He began with the news that it was his 80th birthday and he had decided that as a gift to himself he would prove that he could hike up the mountain. (This, of course, was eight hours and lots of daylight earlier.) He then informed us that he was Arizona's first heart surgeon. He then began to thank us immensely. We let him know that it is our job to help stranded hikers, but that I happened to have food with me because I am diabetic. The next thing he said shocked me just a little bit. Mr. Baker informed me that he had a clinic for diabetics. His clinic provided free dental care and diabetes care for Hispanics in the inner city with diabetes. Mr. Baker went on and on about how his wife must have sent us to save him, then mentioned that his wife had past away many years prior. How amazing that my partner and I would save a man that had a clinic for diabetics!! He was surprised at my ability to handle the stresses of being a Park Ranger and commended me on my perseverance. I ended up having to carry Mr. Baker down the mountain on my back, (we only fell two or three times) which was a tremendous feat for me with my disease and the fact that I had been hiking all day long.

Since Mr. Baker lived just a short walk from the trail, my partner and I took him all the way to his home. Mr. Baker's home was an array of photographs of him posing with many other affluent people; one of which was former U.S. Senator Barry Goldwater. It made me realize what type of man we had just rescued. My partner and I stayed at his home for just a few moments to make sure that Mr.

Baker's health was going to stay stable. I just could not believe that I had just spent the last few hours helping a man that gave a large portion of his life to helping those with diabetes. God had definitely prepared me for that moment, so that I could have the opportunity to help someone that put so much effort into helping others. Little did I know that my weakness would become my strength.

Diabetes is now a strength to me, not a weakness. It is a strength in the fact that I have the opportunity to teach others about proper nutrition since I have to follow a healthy diet in order to survive. It is a strength in the fact that it has taught me to be prepared. It is a strength in the fact hat it gives me the opportunity to overcome obstacles that in the past would have been impossible for a diabetic. I do have many weaknesses, but diabetes is not one of them. I have chosen to conquer diabetes. I have chosen to conquer this disease despite the fact that I was told that I would never grow old, I was told that I would never be police officer, I was told that I would never be a Park Ranger, and I was told that I would never see again after going blind from this devastating disease. I have looked "never" in the eye and I have conquered it. And I am not finished yet. I want to make everyone in this nation aware of this disease that has now become an

133

epidemic. I want to make everyone in this country aware of this disease that is one of the leading causes of blindness here in the United States. I want to make everyone in this country aware of this disease that is devastating our youth. I want awareness in schools, I want awareness in the workplace, and I want awareness in the marketplace where one in every five people surrounding you has this disease. Look around. It is time to become aware. It is time to realize that the next diagnosis could be your own. It is time to open YOUR eyes to diabetes. It is time for this country to no longer be blind to all of us suffering from diabetes.

www.ingramcontent.com/pod-product-compliance
Lightning Source LLC
Chambersburg PA
CBHW031211270326
41931CB00006B/519